Department of Veterans Affairs
Health Services Research & Development Service | Evidence-based Synthesis Program

QUERI

Comparative Effectiveness of Newer Oral Anticoagulants and Standard Anticoagulant Regimens for Thromboprophylaxis in Patients Undergoing Total Hip or Knee Replacement

December 2012

Prepared for:
Department of Veterans Affairs
Veterans Health Administration
Quality Enhancement Research Initiative
Health Services Research & Development Service
Washington, DC 20420

Prepared by:
Evidence-based Synthesis Program (ESP) Center
Durham Veterans Affairs Healthcare System
Durham, NC
John W. Williams Jr., M.D., M.H.Sc., Director

Investigators:
Principal Investigator:
Soheir S. Adam, M.D.

Co-Investigators:
Jennifer R. McDuffie, Ph.D.
Paul F. Lachiewicz, M.D.
Thomas L. Ortel, M.D., Ph.D.
John W. Williams Jr., M.D., M.H.Sc.

Research Associate:
Avishek Nagi, M.S.

Medical Editor:
Liz Wing, M.A.

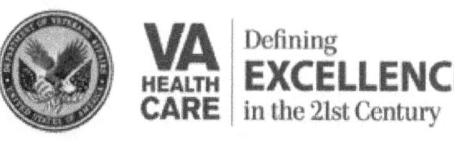

PREFACE

Quality Enhancement Research Initiative's (QUERI's) Evidence-based Synthesis Program (ESP) was established to provide timely and accurate syntheses of targeted healthcare topics of particular importance to Veterans Affairs (VA) managers and policymakers, as they work to improve the health and healthcare of Veterans. The ESP disseminates these reports throughout VA.

QUERI provides funding for four ESP Centers and each Center has an active VA affiliation. The ESP Centers generate evidence syntheses on important clinical practice topics, and these reports help:
- develop clinical policies informed by evidence,
- guide the implementation of effective services to improve patient outcomes and to support VA clinical practice guidelines and performance measures, and
- set the direction for future research to address gaps in clinical knowledge.

In 2009, the ESP Coordinating Center was created to expand the capacity of QUERI Central Office and the four ESP sites by developing and maintaining program processes. In addition, the Center established a Steering Committee comprised of QUERI field-based investigators, VA Patient Care Services, Office of Quality and Performance, and Veterans Integrated Service Networks (VISN) Clinical Management Officers. The Steering Committee provides program oversight, guides strategic planning, coordinates dissemination activities, and develops collaborations with VA leadership to identify new ESP topics of importance to Veterans and the VA healthcare system.

Comments on this evidence report are welcome and can be sent to Nicole Floyd, ESP Coordinating Center Program Manager, at nicole.floyd@va.gov.

Recommended citation: Adam SS, McDuffie JR, Lachiewicz PF, Ortel TL, Williams JW Jr. Comparative Effectiveness of Newer Oral Anticoagulants and Standard Anticoagulant Regimens for Thromboprophylaxis in Patients Undergoing Total Hip or Knee Replacement. VA ESP Project #09-010; 2012.

This report is based on research conducted by the Evidence-based Synthesis Program (ESP) Center located at the Durham VA Medical Center, Durham, NC, funded by the Department of Veterans Affairs, Veterans Health Administration, Office of Research and Development, Health Services Research and Development. The findings and conclusions in this document are those of the author(s) who are responsible for its contents; the findings and conclusions do not necessarily represent the views of the Department of Veterans Affairs or the United States government. Therefore, no statement in this article should be construed as an official position of the Department of Veterans Affairs. Potential conflicts of interest: Dr. Ortel: *Grants*–GlaxoSmithKline, Eisai, Daichi Sankyo, Pfizer, Instrumentation Laboratory; *Consultancy*–Boehringer Ingelheim, Pfizer, Instrumentation Laboratory. No other investigators have any affiliations or financial involvement (e.g., employment, consultancies, honoraria, stock ownership or options, expert testimony, grants or patents received or pending, or royalties) that conflict with material presented in the report. To limit conflict of interest, Dr. Ortel participated in the design and critical review of the report but did not participate in data abstraction or drafting of the report.

TABLE OF CONTENTS

EXECUTIVE SUMMARY
    Background 1
    Methods 2
    Data Synthesis 2
    Rating the Body of Evidence 2
    Peer Review 3
    Results 3
    Recommendations for Future Research 9
    Conclusion 9
    Abbreviations Table 10

INTRODUCTION
    Pharmacological Treatment Options for VTE Thromboprophylaxis 11

METHODS
    Topic Development 13
    Analytic Framework 13
    Search Strategy 14
    Study Selection 14
    Data Abstraction 15
    Quality Assessment 16
    Data Synthesis 16
    Rating the Body of Evidence 17
    Peer Review 18

RESULTS
    Literature Search 19
    Study Characteristics 20
    Participant Characteristics 22
    KQ 1. Comparative effectiveness of newer oral anticoagulants and standard drug classes 23
    KQ 2. Comparative effects of combined pharmacological and mechanical modalities 27
    KQ 3. Comparative efficacy of newer oral anticoagulants 28

SUMMARY AND DISCUSSION
    Summary of Evidence by Key Question 30
    Clinical and Policy Implications 34
    Applicability 36
    Strengths and Limitations 36
    Recommendations for Future Research 36
    Conclusion 37

REFERENCES 38

APPENDIX A	SEARCH STRATEGIES	42
APPENDIX B	EXCLUDED STUDIES	43
APPENDIX C	SAMPLE DATA ABSTRACTION FORM	46
APPENDIX D	CRITERIA USED IN QUALITY ASSESSMENT OF SYSTEMATIC REVIEWS	49
APPENDIX E	PEER REVIEW COMMENTS	52
APPENDIX F	GLOSSARY	56

FIGURES

- Figure 1. Analytic framework for the comparative effectiveness of newer oral anticoagulants 13
- Figure 2. Literature flow diagram 19

TABLES

- Table 1. Summary of the strength of evidence for KQ 1 5
- Table 2. Summary of the strength of evidence for KQ 3 8
- Table 3. Evidence gaps and future research 9
- Table 4. Summary of inclusion and exclusion criteria 15
- Table 5. Characteristics of included systematic reviews 21
- Table 6. Characteristics of patient samples 22
- Table 7. Summary of the strength of evidence for KQ 1 31
- Table 8. Summary of the strength of evidence for KQ 3 33
- Table 9. U.S. guideline recommendations related to specific thromboprophylaxis strategies 35
- Table 10. Evidence gaps and future research 37

EXECUTIVE SUMMARY

BACKGROUND

Venous thromboembolic (VTE) events are important causes of morbidity in elective total hip replacement (THR) and total knee replacement (TKR) procedures. Current guidelines recommend thromboprophylaxis in patients undergoing THR or TKR, although the American Academy of Orthopaedic Surgeons (AAOS) guidelines suggest individual assessment of patients when choosing the specific thromboprophylaxis strategy. Low molecular weight heparin (LMWH) and adjusted-dose warfarin are the most commonly used anticoagulants for thromboprophylaxis in the United States, but a number of other treatment options are available, including unfractionated heparin, aspirin, mechanical devices, and newer oral anticoagulants.

Prior to 1980, rates of symptomatic VTE were 15 to 30 percent. However, improved surgical care and techniques have decreased the rate of symptomatic VTE. A recent analysis that incorporated data from trials and observational studies estimated the contemporary 35-day rate of symptomatic VTE without thromboprophylaxis at 4.3 percent.

Pharmacological thromboprophylaxis for THR or TKR surgery decreases VTE by approximately 50 percent but with the tradeoff of increased bleeding. The risk of bleeding is a concern because bleeding can lead to infections, reoperation, delayed wound healing, and extended hospital stay. The choice of which antithrombotic thus becomes pivotal for balancing the prevention of thromboembolism with the risk of bleeding. Newer oral anticoagulants have been developed with the goal of overcoming the limitations of warfarin and the available parenteral agents. These newer anticoagulants belong to two drug classes, based on their target coagulation protein: factor Xa (FXa) inhibitors and direct thrombin inhibitors (DTIs). These drugs are given as fixed oral doses and have the advantage of a more predictable anticoagulant effect, eliminating the need for monitoring when used for short-term thromboprophylaxis. Disadvantages of newer oral anticoagulants include the lack of specific antidotes to reverse their anticoagulant effect in a timely fashion in case of bleeding, and drug costs.

Given the emerging data on new oral anticoagulants, this report was commissioned by the VA to examine the following key questions (KQs):

KQ 1. For patients undergoing total hip or total knee replacement, what is the comparative effectiveness of newer oral anticoagulants and standard drug classes (low molecular weight heparin, injectable factor Xa inhibitors, unfractionated heparin, warfarin, aspirin) on the incidence of symptomatic, objectively confirmed venous thromboembolism (VTE), other VTE events, total mortality, and bleeding outcomes?

KQ 2. For patients undergoing total hip or total knee replacement, what are the effects of combined pharmacological and mechanical modalities versus pharmacological treatment alone on the incidence of symptomatic, objectively confirmed VTE, other VTE events, total mortality, and bleeding outcomes?

KQ 3. For patients undergoing total hip or total knee replacement, what is the comparative efficacy of individual newer oral anticoagulants on the incidence of symptomatic, objectively confirmed VTE, other VTE events, total mortality, and bleeding outcomes?

METHODS

During the topic development phase of this study, we identified a number of published high-quality systematic reviews that addressed our KQs. We conducted a synthesis of these reviews as they pertained to the KQs and the Veteran population and followed a standard protocol for all steps of this review. We searched MEDLINE® (via PubMed®), Embase®, and the Cochrane Database of Systematic Reviews for systematic review publications comparing the newer oral anticoagulants to other types of anticoagulation (aspirin, warfarin, LMWH, unfractionated heparin, etc.) from January 2009 through September 2012. Our search strategy used the National Library of Medicine's medical subject headings (MeSH) keyword nomenclature and text words for newer oral anticoagulants, the conditions of interest, and validated search terms for systematic reviews.

Using prespecified inclusion and exclusion criteria, two reviewers assessed titles and abstracts for relevance to the KQs. Full-text systematic reviews identified by either reviewer as potentially relevant were retrieved for further review. Select data from published reports were then abstracted into the final abstraction form by a trained reviewer. All data abstractions were confirmed by a second reviewer. We also abstracted data necessary for assessing the quality of systematic reviews, adapted from the AMSTAR criteria. Based on these criteria, systematic reviews were categorized as good, fair, or poor quality. Poor-quality reviews were excluded.

DATA SYNTHESIS

We categorized each systematic review by the key research questions they addressed and critically analyzed them to compare their characteristics, methods, and findings. We summarized the key findings and conclusions from each included review and produced summary tables for comparison across reviews. We prioritized the evidence from these reviews by the quality of methodological designs, more complete drug comparisons, and detailed information about population, specific drug intervention, and definitions of outcomes. In addition to summary measures of relative effects (e.g., risk ratios), we report absolute risk differences in the summary strength of evidence tables. For these estimates, baseline risk for patients treated with LMWH—the common comparator for newer anticoagulants—was estimated for each major outcome as symptomatic deep vein thrombosis (DVT), 9 per 1000 patients; nonfatal pulmonary embolism (PE), 3 per 1000 patients; mortality, 3 per 1000 patients; and major bleeding, 7 per 1000 patients.

Our synthesis focused on identifying patterns in efficacy and safety of the different drugs. To determine the consistency of results and conclusions, we then compared each additional review that addressed the same key question. If findings or conclusions differed importantly across reviews, we analyzed potential reasons for discrepancies such as the primary literature included, inclusion/exclusion criteria, differences in outcome definition, analytic approach, and conflict of interest. Because total hip and knee replacement have distinct primary endpoints, we examined the groups of studies as they pertained to these diagnoses separately.

RATING THE BODY OF EVIDENCE

In addition to rating the quality of individual studies, we evaluated the overall quality of the evidence for each KQ. In brief, this approach requires assessment of four domains: risk of bias, consistency, directness, and precision. For risk of bias, we considered study design using the quality assessments of the primary literature reported in the systematic reviews. We used results from meta-analyses when evaluating consistency, precision, strength of association, and whether publication bias was detected. Optimal information size and consideration of whether the confidence interval crossed the clinical decision threshold for a therapy were also used when evaluating precision.

PEER REVIEW

A draft version of the report was reviewed by technical experts and clinical leadership. A transcript of their comments can be found in the appendix, which elucidates how each comment was considered in the final report.

RESULTS

Our search for systematic reviews (SRs) identified 182 unique citations from a combined search of MEDLINE via PubMed, Embase, the Cochrane Database of Systematic Reviews, and bibliographies of key articles. After applying inclusion and exclusion criteria at both the title-and-abstract and full-text review levels, the final set of articles used in this evidence report consisted of six recently published, high-quality systematic reviews.

All of the SRs compared newer oral anticoagulants with other drug classes used for thromboprophylaxis in THR or TKR (KQ 1), but specific strategies varied. Two SRs used random-effects meta-analyses to compare drug classes as a whole (e.g., FXa inhibitors versus LMWH) while the other four SRs compared individual drugs, some analyzing THR and TKR studies separately. Two of the six SRs compared one newer oral anticoagulant with another (KQ 3) though all results were based on indirect comparisons; i.e., through common comparison with enoxaparin. Only one SR compared a pharmacological agent plus mechanical modality versus pharmacologic prophylaxis alone (KQ 2).

All reviews assessed the quality of included trials, and overall quality was judged to be good. Publication bias was assessed and did not indicate bias that would favor newer oral anticoagulants. Three of the SRs were unfunded and reported no conflicts of interest. One SR was unfunded but did report a conflict of interest for one author. Two SRs were funded by government agencies.

Key Question 1. For patients undergoing total hip or total knee replacement, what is the comparative effectiveness of newer oral anticoagulants and standard drug classes (low molecular weight heparin, injectable factor Xa inhibitors, unfractionated heparin, warfarin, aspirin) on the incidence of symptomatic, objectively confirmed venous thromboembolism (VTE), other VTE events, total mortality, and bleeding outcomes?

Key Points

- For all-cause mortality and nonfatal PE, there were no important differences between oral FXa inhibitors and LMWH (high strength of evidence). Using a base rate of 9 events per 1000 patients with LMWH, FXa inhibitors were associated with lower symptomatic DVT (4 fewer events per 1000 patients; 95% CI, 3 to 6). Overall, FXa inhibitors were associated with an increased risk of major bleeding, but major bleeding did not differ importantly at low to moderate doses (moderate strength of evidence). Based on subgroup analyses, there was not a consistent pattern of differences in treatment effects for THR and TKR.

- There were fewer studies evaluating oral DTIs than oral FXa inhibitors; all trials compared dabigatran with enoxaparin. Although estimates of effect were often imprecise, there were no significant differences between oral DTIs and enoxaparin for any major outcome.
- Neither oral FXa inhibitors nor DTIs have been compared directly with adjusted-dose warfarin, oral antiplatelet drugs, or unfractionated heparin in existing SRs.

FXa inhibitors. Rivaroxaban and apixaban are the most commonly studied FXa inhibitors, and rivaroxaban is the only FXa inhibitor marketed in the United States. The risk of symptomatic DVT was reduced with FXa inhibitors compared with LMWH, while the risks of nonfatal PE and mortality were not significantly different (all high strength of evidence). The estimated absolute risk difference was 4 fewer symptomatic DVT events for each 1000 patients receiving thromboprophylaxis with FXa inhibitors over 5 weeks compared with LMWH. However, these benefits were offset by an increase in major bleeding (moderate strength of evidence). The absolute risk difference was 2 more major bleeding events per 1000 patients receiving thromboprophylaxis with FXa inhibitors over 5 weeks. Higher doses of FXa inhibitors, but not intermediate or low doses, were associated with increased major bleeding. Subgroup analysis by specific drug and type of surgery showed a reduced risk of bleeding with apixaban compared with LMWH in TKR but not in THR; risk of major bleeding with rivaroxaban did not differ significantly for either surgery. No reviews identified trials comparing oral FXa inhibitors with warfarin, unfractionated heparin, or oral antiplatelet agents.

Direct thrombin inhibitors. Dabigatran is the only FDA-approved oral DTI and the only DTI evaluated in existing SRs. Compared with LMWH, dabigatran was not associated with significant differences for any outcome examined. The strength of evidence was low for most outcomes due to few events and imprecise estimates of effect; also, effects on mortality varied substantially across studies. In addition to the major outcomes, a subgroup analysis in one SR found no significant difference between both treatment groups on bleeding requiring rehospitalization. No reviews identified trials comparing oral DTIs with warfarin, unfractionated heparin, or oral antiplatelet agents. Table 1 summarizes the findings and strength of evidence for the effects of newer oral anticoagulant drug classes compared with enoxaparin in patients undergoing THR or TKR surgery.

Comparative Effectiveness of New Oral Anticoagulants for Thromboprophylaxis

Table 1. Summary of the strength of evidence for KQ 1

Outcome	Number of Studies (Subjects)	Study Design/ Quality	Consistency Directness	Precision Publication Bias	Effect Estimate (95% CI)	SOE
FXa vs. LMWH[a]						
Mortality (up to 10 weeks)	11 (22,838)	RCT/Good	Consistent Direct	Precise None detected	OR=0.95 (0.55 to 1.63) RD=0 (2 fewer to 1 more) deaths/1000 patients	High
Symptomatic DVT (up to 5 weeks)	18 (22,877)	RCT/Good	Consistent Direct	Precise None detected	OR=0.46 (0.30 to 0.70) RD=4 fewer (3 to 6 fewer) events/1000 patients	High
Nonfatal PE (up to 5 weeks)	20 (26,998)	RCT/Good	Consistent Direct	Precise None detected	OR=1.07 (0.65 to 1.73) RD=0 (1 fewer to 2 more) events/1000 patients	High
Major bleeding (up to 5 weeks)	21 (31,424)	RCT/Good	Inconsistent Direct	Precise None detected	OR=1.27 (0.98 to 1.65) RD=2 more (0 to 4 more) events/1000 patients	Moderate
LMWH vs. DTI[b]						
Mortality (up to 13 weeks)	4 (10,080)	RCT/Good	Inconsistent Direct	Imprecise None detected	TKR RR=1.06 (0.36 to 3.12) RD=0 (2 fewer to 6 more) events/1000 patients THR RR=1.17 (0.04 to 36.52) RD=0 (3 fewer to 107 more) events/1000 patients	Low
Symptomatic DVT (up to 5 weeks)	4 (10,264)	RCT/Good	Consistent Direct	Imprecise None detected	RR=0.82 (0.17 to 3.99) RD=2 fewer (7 fewer to 27 more) events/1000 patients	Low
Symptomatic PE (up to 5 weeks)	4 (10,264)	RCT/Good	Consistent Direct	Imprecise None detected	OR=0.69 (0.31 to 1.54) RD=1 fewer (2 fewer to 2 more) events/1000 patients	Low
Major bleeding (up to 5 weeks)	4 (10,264)	RCT/Good	Consistent Direct	Imprecise None detected	RR=0.94 (0.58 to 1.52) RD=0 (3 fewer to 3 more) events/1000 patients	Moderate
FXa or DTI vs. other antithrombotics						
All outcomes	0	NA	NA	NA	Not estimable	Insufficient

[a] Data from Neumann, 2012.
[b] Risk ratio data from Ringerike, 2012, and Gómez-Outes, 2012; risk difference calculated; SOE ratings from Sobieraj, 2012.

Notes: Outcomes are short-term; there may be some differences for hip versus knee replacement (different baseline risk and different duration of anticoagulation in existing studies); there is some evidence that FXa inhibitors at higher doses increase risk of bleeding.

Abbreviations: CI=confidence interval; DVT=deep vein thrombosis; DTI=direct thrombin inhibitor; FXa=factor X inhibitor; LMWH=low molecular weight heparin; NA=not applicable; OR=odds ratio; PE=pulmonary embolism; RCT=randomized controlled trial; RD=risk difference; RR=risk ratio; SOE=strength of evidence; THR=total hip replacement; TKR=total knee replacement

Key Question 2. For patients undergoing total hip or total knee replacement, what are the effects of combined pharmacological and mechanical modalities versus pharmacological treatment alone on the incidence of symptomatic, objectively confirmed VTE, other VTE events, total mortality, and bleeding outcomes?

Key Points

- In the included SRs, no studies were identified that compared the combination of newer oral anticoagulants and mechanical thromboprophylaxis with pharmacological treatment alone.
- Few studies compared older antithrombotics (LMWH, oral antiplatelet agents, or unfractionated heparin) combined with mechanical prophylaxis to pharmacological or mechanical prophylaxis alone.
- The strength of evidence is insufficient to determine the comparative effectiveness for combined pharmacological and mechanical prophylaxis compared with pharmacological prophylaxis alone for all major outcomes prioritized for this report.

No reviews identified trials comparing newer oral anticoagulants combined with mechanical prophylaxis to pharmacological prophylaxis alone. Even when considering standard treatments, very little data are available comparing combined-modality thromboprophylaxis and pharmacologic prophylaxis only. One SR found moderate strength of evidence that combined-modality thromboprophylaxis was associated with a decreased risk of overall DVT (including asymptomatic events) compared with pharmacologic prophylaxis alone. The evidence was insufficient for all other outcomes.

Key Question 3. For patients undergoing total hip or total knee replacement, what is the comparative efficacy of individual newer oral anticoagulants on the incidence of symptomatic, objectively confirmed VTE, other VTE events, total mortality, and bleeding outcomes?

Key Points

- No clinical trials directly compared newer oral anticoagulants with each other for thromboprophylaxis of THR or TKR.
- The included SRs did not estimate the comparative efficacy of newer oral anticoagulants for symptomatic DVT, nonfatal PE, all-cause mortality, or surgical site bleeding.
- Based on indirect comparisons, there were few differences between newer oral anticoagulants for the outcomes examined. Rivaroxaban was associated with more major bleeding than apixaban (RR 1.59; 95% CI, 0.84 to 3.02). In contrast, the risk of symptomatic VTE was lower for rivaroxaban than apixaban or dabigatran, but confidence intervals included the possibility of a chance association.

Only indirect comparisons of rivaroxaban, apixaban, and dabigatran were performed through common comparison with LMWH. These comparisons were made for only two of our major outcomes—symptomatic VTE (DVT or PE) and major bleeding. There were no significant differences in treatment effect for symptomatic VTE or major bleeding. Because these indirect comparisons are subject to confounding and the treatment effects were imprecise, we considered the strength of evidence low. Other outcomes reported included clinically relevant bleeding and net clinical endpoints. Rivaroxaban was found to be associated with an increased risk of clinically relevant bleeding, but there was no significant difference in net clinical endpoints (symptomatic VTE, major bleeding, and death). Table 2 summarizes the findings and strength of evidence for between-drug comparisons of newer oral anticoagulants in patients undergoing THR or TKR.

Table 2. Summary of the strength of evidence for KQ 3

Outcome	Number of Studies (Subjects)	Domains Pertaining to SOE			Effect Estimate (95% CI)	SOE
		Study Design/ Quality	Consistency Directness	Precision Publication Bias		
Apixaban, rivaroxaban, dabigatran[a]						
Mortality	NR	NA	NA	NA	Outcome not reported	Insufficient
Symptomatic DVT	NR	NA	NA	NA	Outcome not reported	Insufficient
Nonfatal PE	NR	NA	NA	NA	Outcome not reported	Insufficient
Symptomatic VTE	16 (38,747)	RCT/Good	NA Indirect	Imprecise None detected	Rivaroxaban vs. dabigatran RR=0.68 (0.21 to 2.23) RD=3 fewer (11 fewer to 4 more) events/1000 patients	Low
					Rivaroxaban vs. apixaban RR=0.59 (0.26 to 1.33) RD=4 fewer (9 fewer to 1 more)/1000 patients	Low
					Apixaban vs. dabigatran RR=1.16 (0.31 to 4.28) RD=1 more (7 fewer to 8 more)/1000 patients	Low
Major bleeding	16 (38,747)	RCT/Good	NA Indirect	Imprecise None detected	Rivaroxaban vs. dabigatran RR=1.37 (0.21 to 2.23); RD=4 more (2 fewer to 11 more) events/1000 patients	Low
					Rivaroxaban vs. apixaban RR=1.59 (0.84 to 3.02); RD=5 more (2 fewer to 12 more)/1000 patients	Low
					Apixaban vs. dabigatran RR=1.16 (0.31 to 4.28); RD=0 (8 fewer to 7 more)/1000 patients	Low

[a]Data from Gómez-Outes, 2012.
Abbreviations: DVT=deep vein thrombosis; NA=not applicable; NR=not reported; PE=pulmonary embolism; RCT=randomized controlled trial; RD=risk difference; RR=risk ratio; SOE=strength of evidence; VTE=venous thromboembolism

RECOMMENDATIONS FOR FUTURE RESEARCH

We used a structured framework to identify gaps in evidence and classify why these gaps exist (Table 3).

Table 3. Evidence gaps and future research

Evidence Gap	Reason	Type of Studies to Consider
Absence of direct comparisons between newer anticoagulant drugs	Insufficient information	Multicenter RCTs High-quality network meta-analyses Observational comparative effectiveness studies
Absence of direct comparisons between newer anticoagulants and agents other than LMWH	Insufficient information	Multicenter RCTs Observational comparative effectiveness studies
Absence of comparisons between combined treatment with newer anticoagulants and mechanical thromboprophylaxis to pharmacological or mechanical thromboprophylaxis alone	Insufficient information	Multicenter RCTs Observational comparative effectiveness studies
Adverse effects with long-term use and in usual clinical practice	Insufficient information	Observational studies

Abbreviation: LMWH=low molecular weight heparin; RCT=randomized controlled trial

CONCLUSION

For THR or TKR, the 35-day rate of symptomatic VTE without thromboprophylaxis is estimated to be 4.3 percent. Pharmacological thromboprophylaxis decreases VTE by approximately 50 percent but with the tradeoff of increased bleeding. Newer oral anticoagulants have a more convenient route of administration compared with LMWH, and unlike adjusted dose warfarin, they do not require regular laboratory monitoring. Compared with LMWH, FXa inhibitors are associated with a reduced risk of symptomatic DVT, but mortality and nonfatal PE are not significantly different, and the risk of major bleeding episodes is increased.

There are no available studies on head-to-head comparisons of these novel anticoagulants. Longer clinical experience and direct drug-drug comparisons are needed to better assess the risk-to-benefit ratio of newer oral anticoagulants for surgical thromboprophylaxis. Based on current evidence, newer anticoagulants—particularly FXa inhibitors—are a reasonable option for thromboprophylaxis in patients undergoing total hip replacement or total knee replacement.

ABBREVIATIONS TABLE

CI	confidence interval
DTI	direct thrombin inhibitor
DVT	deep vein thrombosis
FDA	U.S. Food and Drug Administration
FXa	factor Xa inhibitor
INR	international normalized ratio
KQ	key question
LMWH	low molecular weight heparin
MeSH	medical subject heading
NA	not applicable
NR	not reported
OR	odds ratio
PE	pulmonary embolism
RCT	randomized controlled trial
RD	risk difference
RR	risk ratio
SOE	strength of evidence
THR	total hip replacement
TKR	total knee replacement
VA	Department of Veterans Affairs
VHA	Veterans Health Administration
VKA	vitamin K antagonist
VTE	venous thromboembolism

EVIDENCE REPORT

INTRODUCTION

Venous thromboembolic (VTE) events are important causes of morbidity in elective total hip replacement (THR) and total knee replacement (TKR) procedures, which are being performed with increasing frequency in an aging population. Because of the substantial risk of VTE, current guidelines recommend thromboprophylaxis in patients undergoing THR or TKR.[1-3] Low molecular weight heparin (LMWH) and adjusted-dose warfarin are the most commonly used anticoagulants for thromboprophylaxis in the United States,[4] but a number of pharmacological treatment options are available including unfractionated heparin, aspirin, and newer oral anticoagulants. These drug classes differ in practical applications such as a predictable dose-response and the need for laboratory monitoring, oral versus injection administration, dosing frequency, drug-drug interactions, and the availability of an appropriate reversal mechanism in case of over anticoagulation. In addition, mechanical thromboprophylaxis, most frequently used in combination with anticoagulants, is commonly used in the United States.

Risk factors for VTE include venous stasis, endothelial injury, and hypercoagulability. Venous stasis can result from the positioning of the limb, localized postoperative swelling, or limited mobility in the postoperative period.[5,6] Endothelial injury can result from positioning and manipulation of the limb.[5,7] Markers of thrombin generation, indicating hypercoagulability, have been shown to be elevated in total hip arthroplasty.[8] Prior to 1980, rates of symptomatic VTE were 15 to 30 percent. However, changes in surgical care, including earlier ambulation, and changes to surgical technique that are less invasive and possibly less thrombogenic have decreased the rate of symptomatic VTE. A recent analysis that incorporated data from trials and observational studies estimated the contemporary 35-day rate of symptomatic VTE without thromboprophylaxis at 4.3 percent.[1]

Pharmacological thromboprophylaxis for THR or TKR surgery decreases VTE by approximately 50 percent but with the tradeoff of increased bleeding.[9] Surgical procedures may also increase bleeding risk; major bleeding is estimated to occur in 1.5 percent of patients undergoing THR or TKR, even without thromboprophylaxis.[1] The risk of bleeding is a concern because bleeding can lead to infections, reoperation, delayed wound healing, and extended hospital stay.[10] Considering both benefits and risks, guideline panels have issued moderate to strong recommendations for thromboprophylaxis in patients without a contraindication.[1-3] The choice of which antithrombotic thus becomes pivotal for balancing the prevention of thromboembolism with the risk of bleeding.

PHARMACOLOGICAL TREATMENT OPTIONS FOR VTE THROMBOPROPHYLAXIS

The most commonly used anticoagulants are LMWH, fondaparinux, and warfarin.[4,11,12] Unfractionated heparin and antiplatelet agents are rarely used. The efficacy and safety of LMWH for postoperative thromboprophylaxis has been established in more than 30 studies.[3,9,13] LMWH binds to antithrombin and accelerates the inhibition of thrombin and factor X. LMWH has a long half-life, which allows a once-daily dosing schedule and good bioavailability after subcutaneous injection. Disadvantages of LMWH include the need for parenteral administration, high drug cost, and a small risk of heparin-induced thrombocytopenia.[14] Similarly, fondaparinux has good bioavailability when given once daily subcutaneously. Due to the length of the molecule, fondaparinux mainly acts by catalyzing the inhibition of factor Xa (FXa) with essentially no inhibition of thrombin.[15]

For nearly 50 years, warfarin has been successfully used for prophylaxis and treatment of VTE. Warfarin is administered orally once daily and is inexpensive. However, it has several disadvantages, including the need for regular monitoring with international normalized ratio (INR) and numerous interactions with a host of drugs, herbs, and dietary products. Its delayed onset of action can leave patients unprotected in the early postoperative period. In fact, registry data show that surgeons using warfarin are less likely to meet guideline recommendations than with other agents due to failure to meet the target INR.[4]

Newer oral anticoagulants have been developed with the goal to overcome the limitations of warfarin and the available parenteral agents. These new anticoagulants belong to two drug classes, based on their target coagulation protein: FXa inhibitors and direct thrombin inhibitors (DTIs). These are given as fixed oral doses and have the advantage of a more predictable anticoagulant effect, eliminating the need for monitoring when used for short term thromboprophylaxis. Disadvantages of newer oral anticoagulants include drug costs and the lack of specific antidotes to reverse their anticoagulant effect in a timely fashion in case of bleeding. Rivaroxaban, an oral FXa inhibitor, was approved on July 1, 2011, by the U.S. Food and Drug Administration (FDA) for prophylaxis of VTE in adults undergoing orthopedic surgery. Other oral FXa inhibitors that are currently under clinical development include apixaban, edoxaban, and betrixaban. Apixaban is under FDA review for thromboprophylaxis in orthopedic surgery. Dabigatran etexilate is an oral DTI that has been approved in the United States for stroke prevention in atrial fibrillation. Renal excretion is the predominant elimination pathway for dabigatran, with more than 80 percent of systemically available dabigatran eliminated unchanged.[16] Dabigatran has a better drug interaction profile compared with warfarin and is currently under review for FDA approval in patients undergoing elective orthopedic surgery.

Given the emerging data on new oral anticoagulants, this report was commissioned by the VA to assess the comparative effectiveness of newer oral anticoagulants and standard thromboprophylaxis regimens in total hip and knee replacement surgery.

METHODS

TOPIC DEVELOPMENT

This review was commissioned by the VA's Evidence-based Synthesis Program. The topic was nominated after a topic refinement process that included a preliminary review of published peer-reviewed literature, consultation with internal partners and investigators, and consultation with key stakeholders. We further developed and refined the key questions (KQs) based on a preliminary review of published peer-reviewed literature in consultation with VA and non-VA experts.

The final KQs were:

KQ 1. For patients undergoing total hip or total knee replacement, what is the comparative effectiveness of newer oral anticoagulants and standard drug classes (low molecular weight heparin, injectable factor Xa inhibitors, unfractionated heparin, warfarin, aspirin) on the incidence of symptomatic, objectively confirmed venous thromboembolism (VTE), other VTE events, total mortality, and bleeding outcomes?

KQ 2. For patients undergoing total hip or total knee replacement, what are the effects of combined pharmacological and mechanical modalities versus pharmacological treatment alone on the incidence of symptomatic, objectively confirmed VTE, other VTE events, total mortality, and bleeding outcomes?

KQ 3. For patients undergoing total hip or total knee replacement, what is the comparative efficacy of individual newer oral anticoagulants on the incidence of symptomatic, objectively confirmed VTE, other VTE events, total mortality, and bleeding outcomes?

ANALYTIC FRAMEWORK

We followed a standard protocol for all steps of this review; certain methods map to the PRISMA checklist.[17] Our approach was guided by the analytic framework shown in Figure 1.

Figure 1. Analytic framework for the comparative effectiveness of newer oral anticoagulants

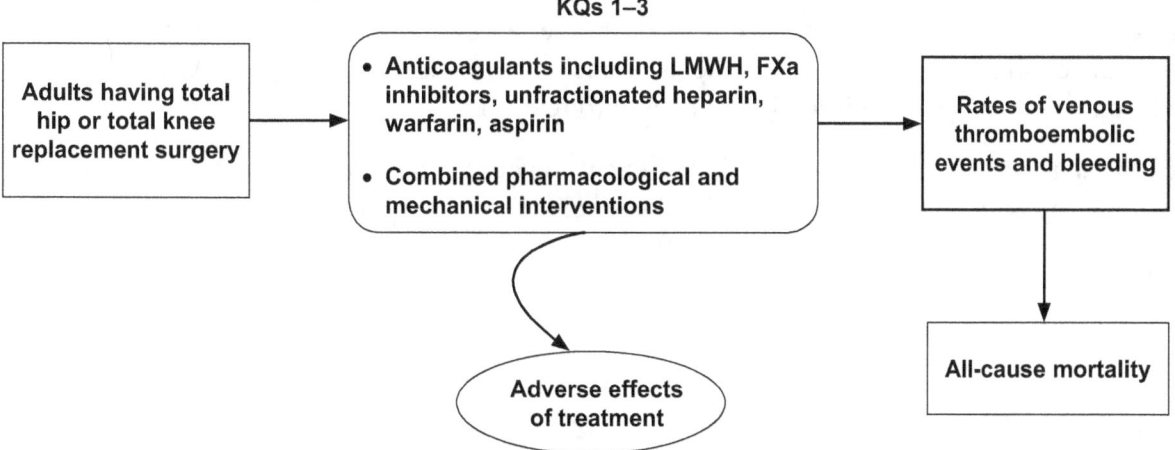

Abbreviations: FXa=factor Xa; KQs=key questions; LMWH=low molecular weight heparin

SEARCH STRATEGY

During the topic development phase of this study, we identified a number of published high-quality systematic reviews that addressed our KQs. We concluded that a synthesis of these reviews as they pertained to the KQs and the Veteran population would be the most effective approach to summarizing the evidence. This approach is particularly useful when different intervention options or outcomes are evaluated in multiple recent reviews and when the audience is policymakers. We searched MEDLINE® (via PubMed®), Embase®, and the Cochrane Database of Systematic Reviews for systematic review publications comparing the newer oral anticoagulants to other types of anticoagulation (aspirin, warfarin, LMWH, unfractionated heparin, etc.) from January 1, 2009, through May 30, 2012. Our search strategy used the National Library of Medicine's medical subject headings (MeSH) keyword nomenclature and text words for newer oral anticoagulants, the conditions of interest, and validated search terms for systematic reviews.[18,19]

Our final search terms included new or novel oral anticoagulants; DTIs, including dabigatran, FXa inhibitors, including edoxaban, rivaroxaban, apixaban, betrixaban, YM150; the MeSH descriptor "orthopedic procedures"; and terms for the specific procedures of interest, total knee replacement or total hip replacement surgery. We limited the search to systematic reviews and meta-analyses and articles published in the English language involving human subjects 18 years of age and older. The full search strategy is provided in Appendix A. We supplemented the electronic searches with a manual search of citations from a set of key systematic reviews[20-23] and clinical guidelines.[1,24] We developed our search strategy in consultation with an experienced search librarian and updated the search during the course of analysis so as not to miss any recent, pertinent reviews; the last update was conducted September 2012. A supplementary search of the primary literature was conducted in September 2012 to identify relevant trials published since May 2012. All citations were imported into an electronic database (DistillerSR; Evidence Partners, Inc., Manotick, ON, Canada) for citation screening.

STUDY SELECTION

Using prespecified inclusion and exclusion criteria, two reviewers assessed titles and abstracts for relevance to the KQs. Full-text systematic reviews identified by either reviewer as potentially relevant were retrieved for further review. Each article retrieved was examined by two reviewers against the eligibility criteria. Disagreements on inclusion, exclusion, or major reason for exclusion were resolved by discussion or by a third reviewer.

The criteria to screen articles for inclusion or exclusion at both the title-and-abstract and full-text screening stages are detailed in Table 4. Studies excluded at the full-text review stage are listed with the reasons for exclusion in Appendix B.

Table 4. Summary of inclusion and exclusion criteria

Study Characteristic	Inclusion Criteria	Exclusion Criteria
Population	Adults (≥18 years) of age undergoing elective orthopedic surgery for total hip or total knee replacement	Pregnant women
Intervention	KQ 1: Newer oral anticoagulants: Direct thrombin inhibitors and factor Xa inhibitors KQ 2: Combined pharmacological and mechanical modalities KQ 3: Newer oral anticoagulants	Newer anticoagulants requiring intravenous or subcutaneous administration
Comparator	KQ 1: Warfarin, low molecular weight heparin, unfractionated heparin, aspirin KQ 2: Pharmacological treatment alone KQ 3: Within-class or between-class comparison with another newer oral anticoagulant	Comparators other than those specified by the KQ inclusion criteria
Outcome	Primary outcomes: Symptomatic, objectively confirmed deep vein thrombosis or pulmonary embolism Secondary outcomes: Major bleeding, surgical-site bleeding, or mortality	No relevant outcomes
Timing	Outcomes reported >1 week postoperatively	Less than 1 week postoperatively
Setting	Inpatient surgical settings	None
Study design	Systematic reviews that evaluated randomized controlled trials (RCTs) or secondary data analysis from an RCT	Not an SR of at least fair or good quality
Publications	English-language only Published from 2009 to present Peer-reviewed article	Non-English language publication Published before 2009

Abbreviations: KQ=key question; RCT=randomized controlled trial

DATA ABSTRACTION

Before general use, the abstraction form templates designed specifically for this report were pilot-tested on a sample of included articles and revised to ensure that all relevant data elements were captured and that there was consistency and reproducibility between abstractors. Select data from published reports were then abstracted into the final abstraction form by a trained reviewer (Appendix C). All data abstractions were confirmed by a second reviewer. Disagreements were resolved by consensus or by obtaining a third reviewer's opinion when consensus could not be reached. We abstracted the following key information for each included study:

- Systematic review design features
    - Databases used in searches and dates of searches
    - Inclusion/exclusion criteria
    - Number of primary studies that apply to each KQ
    - Method of analysis
    - Types of comparisons
    - Tests for heterogeneity
    - Assessment of publication bias

- Characteristics of the included studies
    - Average or range of ages included
    - Average or range of sex distribution
    - Inclusion of Veteran Health Care Facilities
    - Indication for anticoagulation
    - Baseline bleeding risk or factors associated with increased risk (e.g., creatinine >1.5, history of gastrointestinal bleeding), if given
    - Countries included in primary studies
    - Study drug and comparator, route of administration, and dosage
    - Length of treatment and followup duration
    - Funding source

- Results of the systematic review
    - Number of studies and subjects and completion rates
    - Quality of the primary literature and strength of evidence, if given
    - Outcomes (including definition of outcome, if given)
    - Results from subgroup or sensitivity analyses
    - Author conclusions

In addition, we examined included articles for subgroup analyses of particular relevance to the population served by Veterans Health Administration. Data on the inclusion of Veteran Health Care Facilities was not provided at the systematic review level; therefore, we returned to the primary literature to abstract this information.

QUALITY ASSESSMENT

We also abstracted data necessary for assessing the quality of systematic reviews, adapted from the AMSTAR criteria.[25-27] These key quality criteria consist of (1) search methods are adequate for replication and are comprehensive, (2) selection bias is avoided, (3) data are abstracted reliably, (4) characteristics of primary literature are reported and quality is assessed appropriately, (5) results are synthesized using appropriate methods, (6) publication bias is assessed, (7) conflict of interest is reported, and (8) conclusions are supported by results. We supplemented these criteria for studies that used multiple treatment comparisons based on the guidance by Mills et al.[28] Based on these criteria, systematic reviews were categorized as good, fair, or poor quality (Appendix D). Poor-quality reviews were excluded. The criteria were applied for each study by the reviewer abstracting the article; this initial assessment was then overread by a second reviewer. Disagreements were resolved between the two reviewers or, when needed, by arbitration from a third reviewer.

DATA SYNTHESIS

We categorized each systematic review by the key research questions they addressed and critically analyzed them to compare their characteristics, methods, and findings. We summarized the key findings and conclusions from each included review and produced summary tables for comparison across reviews. We prioritized the evidence from these reviews by higher quality of methodological designs, more complete drug comparisons (e.g., by class and drug rather than by drug only), and more detailed information about population, specific drug intervention (e.g., dosage), and definitions of outcomes. In addition to summary measures of relative effects (e.g., risk ratios), we report absolute risk differences in the summary strength of evidence tables. For FXa inhibitors, we used the risk differences reported by Neumann et al.[20] To standardize the reporting of risk differences, which are dependent on the baseline risk of events, we adopted the approach used by Neumann et al. for other drugs. Risk difference was estimated by using the baseline risk from the control group and the risk ratio from the relevant meta-analysis. Baseline risk for patients treated with LMWH, the common comparator for newer anticoagulants, was estimated for each major outcome as symptomatic deep vein thrombosis (DVT), 9 per 1000 patients; nonfatal pulmonary embolism (PE), 3 per 1000 patients; mortality, 3 per 1000 patients; and major bleeding, 7 per 1000 patients.[20]

Our synthesis focused on documenting and identifying patterns in efficacy and safety of the different drugs. To determine the consistency of results and conclusions, we then compared each additional review that addressed the same key question. If findings or conclusions differed importantly across reviews, we analyzed potential reasons for discrepancies such as the primary literature included (both the type of studies and the dates of the searches), review inclusion/exclusion criteria, differences in outcome definition, analytic approach, and conflict of interest.

In the event that our supplemental search of the primary literature identified additional eligible studies, we planned a qualitative summary of these studies to determine if the outcomes observed were consistent with the results from the systematic reviews. However, our search did not identify any additional relevant RCTs.

RATING THE BODY OF EVIDENCE

In addition to rating the quality of individual studies, we evaluated the overall quality of the evidence for each KQ as described in the *Methods Guide for Effectiveness and Comparative Effectiveness Reviews*.[29] In brief, this approach requires assessment of four domains: risk of bias, consistency, directness, and precision. For risk of bias, we considered basic (e.g., RCT) and detailed study design (e.g., adequate randomization) using the quality assessments of the primary literature reported in the systematic reviews. We used results from meta-analyses when evaluating consistency (forest plots, tests for heterogeneity), precision (confidence intervals), strength of association (odds ratio), and whether publication bias was detected (e.g., funnel plots or Begg's test). Optimal information size and consideration of whether the confidence interval crossed the clinical decision threshold for a therapy were also used when evaluating precision.[30]

These domains were considered qualitatively, and a summary rating of high, moderate, low, or insufficient strength of evidence was assigned after discussion by two reviewers. This four-level rating scale consists of the following definitions:

- **High**—Further research is very unlikely to change our confidence on the estimate of effect.
- **Moderate**—Further research is likely to have an important impact on our confidence in the estimate of effect and may change the estimate.
- **Low**—Further research is very likely to have an important impact on our confidence in the estimate of effect and is likely to change the estimate.

- **Insufficient**—Evidence on an outcome is absent or too weak, sparse, or inconsistent to estimate an effect.

When a rating of high, moderate, or low was not possible or was imprudent to make, a grade of insufficient was assigned.[31]

PEER REVIEW

A draft version of the report was reviewed by technical experts and clinical leadership. A transcript of their comments can be found in Appendix E, which elucidates how each comment was considered in the final report.

RESULTS

LITERATURE SEARCH

The flow of articles through the literature search and screening process is illustrated in Figure 2. Our search for systematic reviews (SRs) identified 162 unique citations from a combined search of MEDLINE via PubMed (n=117), Embase (n=42), and the Cochrane Database of Systematic Reviews (n=3). Manual searching of included study bibliographies and review articles added 20 more citations for a total of 182 unique citations. After applying inclusion and exclusion criteria at the title-and-abstract level, 47 full-text articles were retrieved and screened. Of these, 38 were excluded at the full-text screening stage, leaving 9 articles (representing 9 unique studies) for data abstraction. After further review, we excluded three systematic reviews[32-34] because they reviewed only one drug of interest and all of the primary studies included in these systematic reviews were already represented in another, more comprehensive included review. Thus, the final set of articles used in this evidence report comprises six systematic reviews.

Appendix B provides a complete listing of published articles excluded at the full-text screening stage, with reasons for exclusion. We did not search www.clinicaltrials.gov for randomized controlled trials (RCTs) currently underway, as we relied on methods in the included systematic reviews to ascertain publication bias. We grouped the studies by key question (Figure 2).

Figure 2. Literature flow diagram

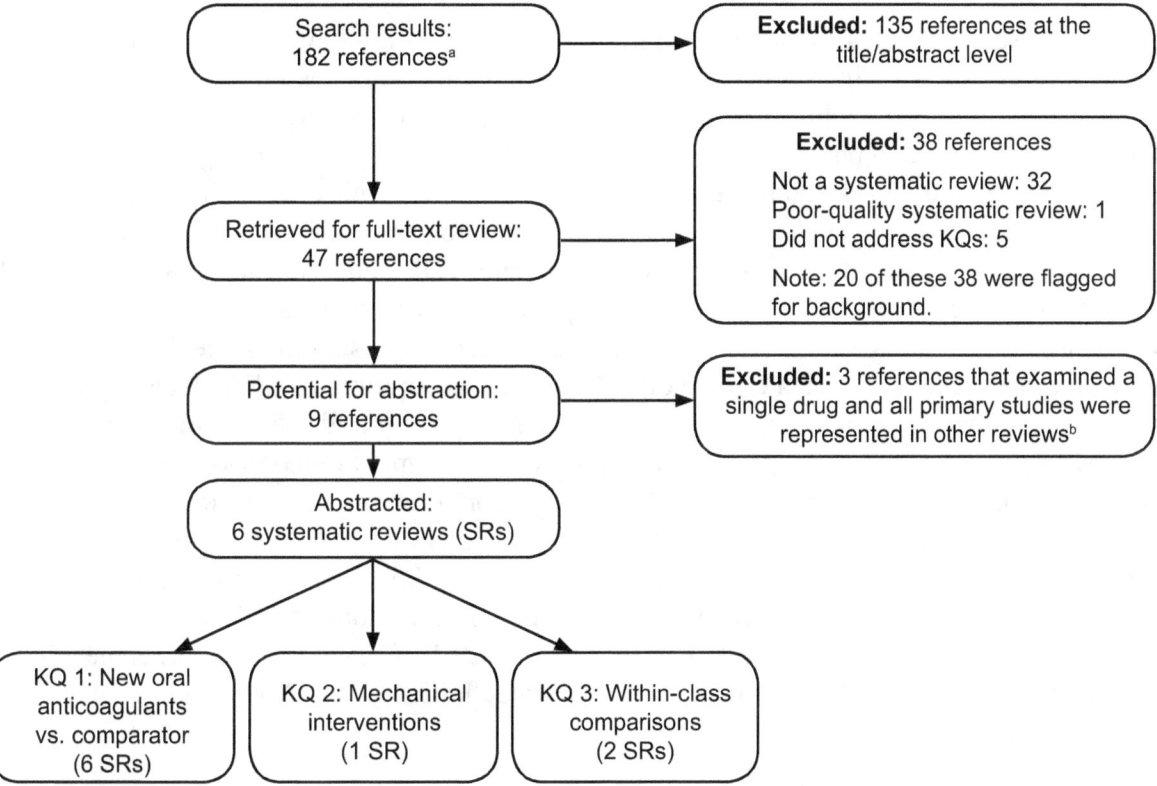

[a]Search results for systematic reviews from PubMed (117), Embase (42), Cochrane (3), previous database (14), and manual (6) were combined.
[b]Cao, 2010; Huang, 2011; and Turun, 2011.
Note: The reference list of this report includes additional references cited for background and methods plus Web sites relevant to the key questions.
Abbreviations: KQ=key question; SR=systematic review

STUDY CHARACTERISTICS

We identified six recent, good-quality SRs[9,20-23,35] that were relevant to our KQs (Table 5). All of the SRs compared newer oral anticoagulants with other drug classes used for thromboprophylaxis in THR or TKR (KQ 1), although one considered only safety outcomes such as major bleeding.[35] Two of the six SRs compared one newer oral anticoagulant with another (KQ 3) though all results were based on indirect comparisons; i.e., through common comparison with enoxaparin.[21,23] Only one SR[9] compared a pharmacological agent plus mechanical modality versus mechanical modality alone (KQ 2). Five of the six SRs included trials examining thromboprophylaxis for both THR and TKR, while one also included hip fracture surgery.[9] Characteristics of the SRs are summarized in Table 5; detailed quality assessments are presented in Appendix D.

Search dates ranged from May 2009 to December 2011. All literature search strategies included MEDLINE, and all but one[21] included some aspect of the Cochrane Library. Other databases or sources of information were meeting abstracts (5), Embase (3), regulatory Web sites (4), clinical trial registries (3), and the Center for Reviews and Dissemination (1). Four studies[9,20-22] also involved a manual search of the bibliographies of exemplary primary articles. The searches were limited only to RCTs in four of the SRs. One included SRs,[22] and one included observational studies of more than 750 subjects[9] in addition to RCTs. Language limits were used in only two of the studies.

All reviews assessed the quality of included trials. Overall trial quality was judged to be good, with the most common quality problems being unclear allocation concealment and incomplete reporting of outcome data. Publication bias was assessed most commonly with funnel plots, which did not indicate any publication bias that would favor newer oral anticoagulants. All studies conducted random-effects meta-analyses, but specific strategies varied. Two SRs compared drug classes as a whole (for example, FXa inhibitors versus LMWH[9,20]), while the other four SRs compared individual drugs, some analyzing THR and TKR studies separately. All of the SRs performed meta-analysis using direct comparisons, and two also provided indirect comparisons.[21,23] Every SR except one[21] evaluated major bleeding using the same definition: bleeding that was fatal, involved a critical organ, required reoperation, or where bleeding was associated with a fall in hemoglobin level of at least 2 g/dL or required infusion of 2 or more units of whole blood or packed cells. Our other prespecified primary outcomes—all-cause mortality, symptomatic DVT, and nonfatal PE—were reported in three of the SRs.[9,20,22] It was difficult to evaluate the other SRs[21,23,35] due to the individuality of the definitions given for the outcomes reported, many of which were composite outcomes. For example, in the study by Loke et al.,[21] the authors state the composite primary outcome as "total VTE" and define it as "DVT, non-fatal PE and all-cause mortality" (emphasis added). The study also reports bleeding as a combination of major bleeding (using the standard definition given above) and "clinically relevant non-major bleeding."

Three of the SRs were unfunded and reported no conflicts of interest.[21,23,35] One SR was unfunded but did report a conflict of interest for one author.[20] Two SRs were funded by government agencies.[9,22]

Table 5. Characteristics of included systematic reviews

Study	Neumann, 2012[20]	Sobieraj, 2012[9]	Gómez-Outes, 2012[23]	Loke, 2011[21]	Ringerike, 2011[22]	Alves, 2011[35]
Quality	Good	Good	Good	Good	Good	Good
Applicable KQ[a]	KQ 1	KQs 1, 2	KQs 1, 3	KQs 1, 3	KQ 1	KQ 1 (safety only)
Orthopedic procedures	THR, TKR	THR, TKR, HFS	THR, TKR	THR, TKR	THR, TKR	THR, TKR
Intervention and comparator for direct comparisons	As drug classes: - FXa vs. LMWH (LMWH/warfarin in one of 22 studies)	As drug classes: - FXa vs. LMWH - DTI vs. LMWH - DTI vs. UFH	As individual drugs vs. LMWH: - Apixaban - Dabigatran - Rivaroxaban	As individual drugs vs. LMWH: - Dabigatran - Rivaroxaban	As individual drugs vs. LMWH: - Dabigatran - Rivaroxaban	As individual drugs vs. LMWH: - Apixaban - Rivaroxaban
Databases	MEDLINE, Embase, CCRCT, meeting abstracts	MEDLINE, CCRCT, Scopus, clinical trial registries, meeting abstracts, regulatory Web sites	MEDLINE, CCRCT, clinical trial registries, meeting abstracts, regulatory Web sites	MEDLINE, Embase, clinical trial registries, regulatory Web sites	MEDLINE, Embase, Cochrane Library and Center for Reviews and Dissemination	MEDLINE, Cochrane Library, meeting abstracts, regulatory Web sites
Search date	December 2011	May 2011	April 2011	May 2009	September 2010	June 2011
Language limits	None	None	None	None	English, Scandinavian	None
Study designs	RCTs	RCTs, observational if more than 750 subjects	RCTs	RCTs	RCTs, SRs	RCTs
Analytic approach	Meta-analysis, direct, subgroup by dosage	Meta-analysis, direct, indirect, network MA	Meta-analysis, direct, indirect, subgroup by surgery type	Meta-analysis, direct, indirect, subgroup by protocol	Meta-analysis, subgroup by type of surgery	Meta-analysis, direct, subgroup by surgery type
Major outcomes analyzed (included in most studies)	Mortality, symptomatic DVT, nonfatal PE, major bleeding	Mortality, symptomatic DVT, nonfatal PE, major bleeding	Symptomatic DVT, nonfatal PE, major bleeding	None included	Mortality, symptomatic DVT, nonfatal PE, major bleeding	Major bleeding
Other outcomes of interest	Intracranial bleeding, bleeding leading to reoperation	Symptomatic VTE, major VTE, PE, surgical site bleeding, readmission	Total VTE or mortality, symptomatic VTE, clinically relevant bleeding	Total VTE (mortality + DVT + nonfatal PE), bleeding (major + clinically relevant nonmajor)	None	Safety variables: Other types of bleeding, adverse events
Source of funding	None	Government	None	None	Government	None
Conflict of interest?	Yes, disclosed	No	No	No	NR	No

[a] KQ 1=between-class comparisons; KQ 2=combined pharmacological and mechanical vs. pharmacological monotherapy; KQ 3=within-class comparisons of newer oral anticoagulants, all of which are indirect via an LWMH

Abbreviations: CCRCT=Cochrane Central Registry of Controlled Trials; CINAHL=Cumulative Index of Nursing and Allied Health Literature; COI=conflict of interest; DTI=direct thrombin inhibitor; DVT=deep vein thrombosis; FXa=factor Xa inhibitor; HFS=hip fracture surgery; KQ=key question; LMWH=low molecular weight heparin; MA=meta-analysis; NR=not reported; PE=pulmonary embolism; RCT=randomized controlled trial; SR=systematic review; THR=total hip replacement; TKR=total knee replacement; UFH=unfractionated heparin; VTE=venous thromboembolism

PARTICIPANT CHARACTERISTICS

Information on the populations studied was very limited in all of the included SRs (Table 6). The number of primary articles included ranged from 5 to 45; total sample size ranged from just over 19,000 to almost 240,000, but two articles did not report the total number of subjects. Females made up approximately 50 to 75 percent of the population when reported. Mean age ranged from 55 to 68 years in the 5 studies reporting age. Weight or body mass index was reported in four studies and indicated most subjects were moderately overweight to slightly obese. Risk factors for VTE were limited to a prior history of VTE (two studies) or history of cancer (one study); only a small proportion of patients had one of these risk factors. No other risk profiles or population characteristics were reported, and no study reported whether or not Veterans were included in the sample. However, our review of the primary studies found that no studies specifically included Veterans or were conducted at VA medical centers.

Table 6. Characteristics of patient samples

Study	Neumann, 2012[20]	Sobieraj, 2012[9]	Gómez-Outes, 2012[23]	Loke, 2011[21]	Ringerike, 2011[22]	Alves, 2011[35]
Studies (N patients)[a]	22 (32,159)	45 (36,152)	16 (38,747)	9 (19,218)	5 (NR)	12 (28,483)
Female (% range)	44.6 to 72.5	RCTs 36.05–84.1% observational 63–65%	50 to 74	55 to 70	NR[b]	51 to 71
Mean age (range)	57.8 to 67.6	RCTs 52.4 to 78.3; observational 66.4 to 71	61 to 68	63.2 to 67.7	NR[b]	60.6 to 67.6
Weight (kg range)	26.5 to 32.7[c]	RCTs 64.2 to 89 kg; observational NR	75 to 89	76 to 89	NR	NR
Veterans?	No	No	No	No	No	No
Risk factors: History of VTE	NR	0 to 14.5%	1 to 4% (9 studies)	NR	NR	NR
History of cancer		0 to 12.4%				
Risk factors[d]	NR	NR	NR	NR	NR	NR

[a]Numbers are for RCTs, with the exception of Ringerike et al., which reviewed three RCTs and two SRs. Sobieraj et al. also reviewed three observational studies including over 239,000 participants.
[b]Ringerike et al. did not give demographics on study populations but did give national statistics on who had these surgeries performed in Sweden: average age is 69.1 and 69.4 yrs and % female is 68.4 and 67.4% on average for THR and TKR, respectively.
[c]Value is in BMI units (kg/m^2).
[d]Risk factors sought were prior gastrointestinal bleeding, anemia, chronic kidney disease, and diabetes mellitus.
Abbreviations: kg=kilogram; NR=not reported; RCT=randomized controlled trial; VTE=venous thromboembolism

KEY QUESTION 1. For patients undergoing total hip or total knee replacement, what is the comparative effectiveness of newer oral anticoagulants and standard drug classes (low molecular weight heparin, injectable FXa inhibitors, unfractionated heparin, warfarin, aspirin) on the incidence of symptomatic, objectively confirmed venous thromboembolism (VTE), other VTE events, total mortality, and bleeding outcomes?

Key Points

- For all-cause mortality and nonfatal PE, there were no important differences between oral FXa inhibitors and LMWH (high strength of evidence). Using a base rate of 9 events per 1000 patients with LMWH, FXa inhibitors were associated with lower symptomatic DVT (4 fewer events per 1000 patients; 95% CI, 3 to 6). Overall, FXa inhibitors were associated with an increased risk of major bleeding, but major bleeding did not differ importantly at low to moderate doses (moderate strength of evidence). Based on subgroup analyses, there was not a consistent pattern of differences in treatment effects for THR and TKR.
- There were fewer studies evaluating oral DTIs than oral FXa inhibitors; all trials compared dabigatran with enoxaparin. Although estimates of effect were often imprecise, there were no significant differences between oral DTIs and enoxaparin for any major outcome.
- Neither oral FXa inhibitors nor DTIs have been compared directly with adjusted-dose warfarin, oral antiplatelet drugs, or unfractionated heparin in existing SRs.

We identified six good-quality SRs[9,20-23,35] that evaluated thromboprophylaxis using newer oral anticoagulants versus LMWH. For each comparison, we focus our discussion on the review having the most recent search date and comprehensive analysis, and which reported our prespecified outcomes of interest. Other reviews are described briefly when findings differed importantly or additional analyses provided relevant results.

Effects of Oral FXa Inhibitors Compared With Low Molecular Weight Heparin

A good-quality SR[20] (search date December 2011) included 22 RCTs and a total of 32,159 patients that compared FXa inhibitors with LMWH for surgical thromboprophylaxis. Eleven of the included studies were on hip replacement, 10 were on knee replacement, and 1 was on either procedure. FXa inhibitors included apixaban (four studies), rivaroxaban (eight studies), edoxaban (four studies), YM150 (two studies), and LY1517717, TAK442, razaxaban, and betrixaban (one study each). Of these drugs, only rivaroxaban is currently available in the United States. In the majority of trials, the European-approved dose of enoxaparin, 40 mg daily, was the comparator instead of the U.S.-approved dose, 30 mg twice daily. The duration of thromboprophylaxis was 14 days or less in all but 4 trials. Patients were followed for less than 14 days in 9 trials, 30 to 70 days in 12 trials, and up to 90 days in one trial. In addition to a random-effects meta-analysis of drug class comparisons, this sophisticated review performed a multiple-treatment-comparison meta-analysis to evaluate effects of FXa dose, and sensitivity analyses to examine the effects of missing outcomes. Pooled estimates of effect were presented as summary odds ratios and summary risk differences. In addition, risk differences were estimated by applying the relative risk reduction from meta-analysis to the baseline risk estimated from a large cohort study.

This SR by Neumann et al.[20] found high strength of evidence suggesting no important difference between oral FXa inhibitors and LMWH for all-cause mortality (OR 0.95; 95% CI, 0.55 to 1.63; I^2=43%) and nonfatal PE (OR 1.07; CI, 0.65 to 1.73; I^2=35%) in patients undergoing THR or TKR. However, high strength of evidence indicated that the risk of symptomatic DVT is decreased by 4 events for every 1000 patients treated using FXa thromboprophylaxis compared with LMWH (OR 0.46; CI, 0.30 to 0.70; I^2=0%). There was moderate strength of evidence because of inconsistency, suggesting that the risk of major bleeding may be increased with oral FXa inhibitors compared with LMWH (OR 1.27; CI, 0.98 to 1.65; I^2=55%). This finding represents an increase of 2 major bleeding events per 1000 patients treated with FXa, for 1 to 5 weeks compared with LMWH. The pooled effect estimate of bleeding that led to reoperation also was increased (OR 1.62; CI, 0.82 to 3.19; I^2=1%), but the confidence interval included the possibility of a chance association.

In a subgroup analysis, higher doses of FXa inhibitors, but not intermediate or lower doses, were associated with increased risk of bleeding (OR 2.50; 95% CI, 1.38 to 4.53; p=0.02). The authors did not report the drug doses used for this subgroup analysis. Total daily doses were reported for the primary studies and ranged from 5 to 20 mg for apixaban and 5 to 60 mg for rivaroxaban. In an analysis that adjusted for FXa dose, there was no significant difference in thrombotic or bleeding outcomes for different FXa inhibitors. Sensitivity analyses that accounted for missing outcomes did not differ appreciably from the main analyses. Thus this SR concluded that while there is no important difference between low-dose oral FXa inhibitors and LMWH for the outcomes of all-cause mortality, nonfatal PE, and major bleeding, there is a small absolute reduction in symptomatic DVT events (4 fewer events per 1000 patients treated). However, most studies included in this SR reported bleeding as a composite outcome and did not include details; this introduces uncertainty about the importance of the reported bleeding events. Other limitations of the included trials in this SR were (1) missing outcomes for 3 to 41 percent of randomized patients, (2) the short duration of followup in many trials, (3) the nonstandard dosing of enoxaparin, and (4) the short duration of prophylaxis in patients undergoing THR.

The other SRs[9,21-23,35] were generally in agreement with the results and conclusions of Neumann et al. Where disagreements occurred, they were mainly due to different outcomes (e.g., composite outcomes), differences in approach to data analysis (separate analyses for each drug), and fewer included studies due to earlier search dates and more restrictive inclusion criteria (e.g., only FDA-approved drugs). Also, most SRs reported on outcomes by individual new oral anticoagulants, whereas those by Neumann et al. and Sobieraj et al. reported on outcomes by drug class.

We summarize below the notable findings from these other SRs:

- In a good-quality review[23] that separately analyzed the effects of apixaban (4 trials) and rivaroxaban (8 trials), both drugs were associated with lower symptomatic DVT than enoxaparin (apixaban, RR 0.41; 95% CI, 0.18 to 0.95, and rivaroxaban, RR 0.40; CI, 0.22 to 0.72). Symptomatic VTE (DVT or PE) was decreased with rivaroxaban (RR 0.48; CI, 0.31 to 0.75; I^2=5%) but not apixaban (RR 0.82; CI, 0.41 to 1.64; I^2=40%). All-cause mortality was not reported as a separate outcome. Symptomatic PE and major bleeding did not differ significantly from LMWH, but confidence intervals for these estimates were wide and included the potential for clinically important differences. Notably, to increase the consistency of outcome definitions and results, major bleeding rates for the RECORD studies of rivaroxaban[36-39] were analyzed using data reported to the FDA—a definition that included wound bleeding. Subgroup analyses showed no differences in treatment effect by type of surgery (THR vs. TKR) for symptomatic VTE or clinically relevant bleeding.

- In a review limited by the exclusion of rivaroxaban,[9] the pooled effect from four RCTs comparing LMWH with FXa inhibitors did not show a significant difference in major bleeding leading to reoperation (OR 0.67; 95% CI, 0.28 to 1.61).
- In a review limited by the exclusion of apixaban,[21] the risk of hemorrhage (major and clinically relevant nonmajor bleeding) did not differ significantly for rivaroxaban compared with LMWH (RR 1.26; 95% CI, 0.94 to 1.69; I^2=28%). Hemorrhage was defined as major bleeding leading to death, reoperation, blood transfusion of two or more units, a drop in hemoglobin level of more than two g/dL, or bleeding into a critical organ. In contrast to the review by Gómez-Outes et al., published rates of bleeding rather than rates reported to the FDA (that included wound bleeding) were used for these analyses.
- A report on adverse outcomes by type of surgery compared two oral FXa inhibitors with enoxaparin.[35] There was a lower risk of major bleeding with apixaban compared with LMWH in TKR (RR 0.56; 95% CI, 0.32 to 0.96) but not in THR (RR 1.22; 95% CI, 0.65 to 2.26). Major bleeding events were not different with rivaroxaban treatment compared with LMWH in both types of surgeries. Subgroup analysis showed an increased risk of bleeding with the 30-mg twice-daily dosing regimen of LMWH compared with the 40-mg once-daily dose.

Effects of Direct Thrombin Inhibitors Compared with Low Molecular Weight Heparin

Only four SRs[9,21-23] included comparisons of dabigatran—the only available DTI—with standard thromboprophylaxis using LMWH. A good-quality SR (search date April 2011) included 4 trials involving 12,897 patients that compared dabigatran with enoxaparin for thromboprophylaxis of THR or TKR.[23] The surgical procedure was THR and TKR in two trials each. In three trials, the comparator was enoxaparin at 40 mg daily, and in one trial the dose was 30 mg twice daily. The duration of thromboprophylaxis was 15 days or less in the two TKR studies and 28 to 35 days in the two THR studies. The duration of followup was approximately 3 months. Three studies used a three-arm design; the dabigatran 150 mg and dabigatran 220 mg treatment arms were combined for meta-analysis. The two-arm trial evaluated dabigatran 220 mg, a dose that is not approved by the FDA. All-cause mortality was not reported as a separate outcome.

In a random-effects meta-analysis, the risk of symptomatic PE (RR 0.69; 95% CI, 0.31 to 1.54; I^2=NR) and symptomatic DVT (RR 0.82; CI, 0.17 to 3.99; I^2=NR) did not differ between dabigatran and enoxaparin.[23] Similarly, there was no statistically significant difference in symptomatic VTE (DVT and PE), but treatment effects differed substantially across studies (I^2=73%). Clinically relevant bleeding events (major bleeding and clinically relevant nonmajor bleeding) were not different with dabigatran treatment (RR 0.94; CI, 0.58 to 1.52; p=0.79). In subgroup analyses, there was no statistically significant interaction between type of surgery and effects on symptomatic VTE or clinically relevant bleeding.

Three other SRs[9,21,22] reported additional outcomes, including mortality, major bleeding, and bleeding leading to rehospitalization, summarized below:

- The SR by Ringerike et al.[22] included an additional study (BISTRO-II)[40] of patients undergoing either THR or TKR, but anticoagulation was given for 7 days only. The SR by Sobieraj et al.[9] evaluated an injectable DTI (desirudin) but did not include the most recent trial of oral DTI,[40] which was also omitted in the SR by Loke et al.[21] Despite these differences in approach, mortality did not differ significantly for DTIs compared with enoxaparin in any of these analyses. Consistent with the findings by Gómez-Outes et al.[23] for clinically relevant bleeding, major bleeding did not differ between drug classes when analyzed by surgical procedure[22] or in aggregate.[9,21]
- Sobieraj et al.[9] found no significant difference between LMWH and dabigatran for bleeding leading to rehospitalization (RR 1.27; 95% CI, 0.43 to 3.75; moderate strength of evidence).

Other Comparisons of Interest

Only one good-quality SR by Sobieraj et al.[9] (search date May 2011) addressed drug class comparisons between older antithrombotics. We summarize results for key drug class comparisons and outcomes below.

Low molecular weight heparin versus vitamin K antagonists. Sobieraj et al.[9] reported on the comparative effects of LMWH thromboprophylaxis versus adjusted-dose warfarin. LMWHs included enoxaparin (30 mg every 12 hours) and logiparin. Other details such as duration of treatment and duration of followup were not reported uniformly for the included trials. Depending on outcomes, 3 to 7 trials were included in the meta-analyses. There was no significant difference in mortality (OR 0.79; 95% CI, 0.42 to 1.50; $I^2=0\%$), nonfatal PE (OR 1.00; CI, 0.20 to 4.95; $I^2=NR$), or symptomatic DVT (OR 0.87; CI, 0.61 to 1.24; $I^2=28.4\%$). The risk of major bleeding was significantly higher in the LMWH treatment group (OR 1.92; CI, 1.27 to 2.91; $I^2=0$; high strength of evidence).

Oral FXa inhibitors versus unfractionated heparin. Sobieraj et al.[9] reported on the comparative effects of oral FXa inhibitors versus unfractionated heparin. There were no RCTs comparing oral or injectable FXa inhibitors with unfractionated heparin. One observational study compared an injectable FXa inhibitor (fondaparinux) with unfractionated heparin; drug doses were not reported. The injectable FXa inhibitor was associated with lower mortality compared with unfractionated heparin. The risk of major bleeding was found to be increased in the unfractionated heparin treatment group compared with the injectable FXa inhibitor group (OR 1.27; 95% CI, 1.06 to 1.52). Effects on symptomatic DVT and nonfatal PE were not reported.

Low molecular weight heparin versus oral antiplatelet agents. Sobieraj et al.[9] reported on the comparative effects of LMWH versus oral antiplatelet agents but identified no studies comparing these drug classes.

Antiplatelet agents versus vitamin K antagonists. Sobieraj et al.[9] reported on the comparative effects of antiplatelet agents versus vitamin K antagonists, identifying a single RCT. Among patients undergoing hip fracture surgery, the risk of mortality was similar in both treatment arms (RR 0.98; 95% CI, 0.32 to 3.05). Nonfatal PE was evaluated, but there were no events in either treatment arm. The risk of major bleeding was also reported in this trial and did not show a statistically significant difference (RR 0.20; CI 0.03 to 1.23). In addition to this RCT, two observational studies compared aspirin prophylaxis with vitamin K antagonists in patients undergoing THR or TKR. One study showed higher mortality with aspirin prophylaxis (0.3 percent vs. 0 percent; p=0.013); the other study found no significant difference in mortality. There were no reports on symptomatic DVT or symptomatic VTE.

KEY QUESTION 2. For patients undergoing total hip or total knee replacement, what are the effects of combined pharmacological and mechanical modalities versus pharmacological treatment alone on the incidence of symptomatic, objectively confirmed VTE, other VTE events, total mortality, and bleeding outcomes?

Key Points

- In the included SRs, no studies were identified that compared the combination of newer oral anticoagulants and mechanical thromboprophylaxis with pharmacological treatment alone.
- Few studies have compared older antithrombotics (LMWH, oral antiplatelet agents, or unfractionated heparin) combined with mechanical prophylaxis to pharmacological or mechanical prophylaxis alone.
- The strength of evidence is insufficient to determine the comparative effectiveness for combined pharmacological and mechanical prophylaxis compared with pharmacological prophylaxis alone for all major outcomes prioritized for this report.

One good-quality SR[9] (search date May 2011) included 6 trials and a total of 995 patients that compared a combined-modality thromboprophylaxis (pharmacological and mechanical agents) with a single modality and found a paucity of data. Four of the included studies were on hip replacement, one was on knee replacement, and one included both surgeries. No trial evaluated the combination of a newer oral anticoagulant together with mechanical prophylaxis. Combination treatments included LMWH, aspirin, or unfractionated heparin together with mechanical prophylaxis. Of the six trials, the comparator was pharmacologic prophylaxis alone (4 trials), mechanical prophylaxis alone (1 trial), and both pharmacological and mechanical comparators (1 trial). Duration of followup ranged from the postoperative period to 90 days.

Three trials reported effects on mortality, but treatment effects were not pooled. Two of these trials had no mortality events; the third trial comparing the combination of aspirin plus pneumatic compression to aspirin alone found no effects on mortality (OR 7.72; 95% CI, 0.15 to 389.59), but the trial was underpowered for clinically significant differences. Two trials evaluated the effects on nonfatal PE, but there were no events in either trial. A single older trial evaluated the effects of sequential unfractionated heparin for 3 days, then aspirin together with a venous foot pump versus sequential pharmacologic prophylaxis alone or a venous foot pump alone. The combined modality had a lower risk of symptomatic DVT compared with pharmacologic prophylaxis only (RR 0.14; 95% CI, 0.01 to 1.42), but there were few events, and the confidence interval included no effect. Only one trial reported the effects of combined thromboprophylaxis (aspirin plus venous foot pump) compared with aspirin alone for major bleeding. However, there were no major bleeding events in either treatment arm. The authors concluded that there was insufficient evidence for all outcomes when comparing pharmacologic plus mechanical prophylaxis to pharmacologic prophylaxis alone, with the exception of overall DVT (including asymptomatic DVT). For overall DVT, combined treatment was more effective than pharmacologic prophylaxis alone.

KEY QUESTION 3. For patients undergoing total hip or total knee replacement, what is the comparative efficacy of individual newer oral anticoagulants on the incidence of symptomatic, objectively confirmed VTE, other VTE events, total mortality, and bleeding outcomes?

Key Points

- No clinical trials directly compared newer oral anticoagulants with each other for thromboprophylaxis of TKR or THR.
- The included SRs did not estimate the comparative efficacy of newer oral anticoagulants for symptomatic DVT, nonfatal PE, all-cause mortality, or surgical site bleeding.
- Based on indirect comparisons, there were few differences between newer oral anticoagulants for the outcomes examined. Rivaroxaban was associated with more major bleeding than apixaban (RR 1.59; 95% CI, 0.84 to 3.02). In contrast, the risk of symptomatic VTE was lower for rivaroxaban than apixaban or dabigatran, but confidence intervals included the possibility of a chance association.

In the absence of direct comparisons between the newer oral anticoagulants, two good-quality SRs used indirect comparisons[21,23] to analyze these drugs.

A good-quality comprehensive review[23] (search date April 2011) evaluated apixaban (4 trials), dabigatran (4 trials), and rivaroxaban (8 trials) against a common comparator (enoxaparin). These indirect comparisons utilized pooled risk ratios and yielded an unbiased estimate of effect "when there is no interaction between covariates defining subgroups of patients (reflected, for instance, in different inclusion criteria in different studies) and the magnitude of the treatment effect."[41] Of the 16 trials (total of 38,747 patients), 8 were of total hip replacement and 8 of total knee replacement. Outcomes reported in the indirect comparisons included symptomatic venous thromboembolism (DVT or PE), clinically relevant bleeding (major bleeding or clinically relevant nonmajor bleeding), major bleeding, and a net clinical endpoint—defined as a composite of symptomatic VTE, major bleeding, and all-cause death. Overall, the primary trials were rated low risk of bias. Individual drug comparisons across these 4 outcomes (12 comparisons) showed only one statistically significant difference: rivaroxaban resulted in more clinically relevant bleeding compared with apixaban (RR 1.52; 95% CI, 1.19 to 1.95). The risk of major bleeding was also increased with rivaroxaban compared with apixaban (RR 1.59; CI, 0.84 to 3.02), but the difference was not statistically significant. Rivaroxaban was associated with lowest risk of symptomatic VTE compared with dabigatran (RR 0.68; CI, 0.21 to 2.23) and apixaban (RR 0.59; CI, 0.26 to 1.33), but neither comparison was statistically significant. Overall, differences in the number of VTE events were offset by the number of major bleeding episodes. Thus, there was no difference on the net clinical endpoint among apixaban, dabigatran, and rivaroxaban. The review concluded that "higher efficacy of new anticoagulants was generally associated with higher bleeding tendency. The new anticoagulants did not differ significantly for efficacy and safety."[23]

The other SR provided few additional relevant findings. Similar to the review described above, Loke et al.[21] (search date May 2009) used indirect analysis methods but excluded studies of apixaban, yielding a less informative analysis. In addition, a dabigatran trial published after 2009 and three rivaroxaban studies were excluded due to more restrictive eligibility criteria. Despite these differences, findings regarding rivaroxaban compared with dabigatran were generally similar. The authors concluded that rivaroxaban was superior to dabigatran in preventing VTE (RR 0.50; 95% CI, 0.37 to 0.68) although with an increased risk of bleeding (RR 1.14; CI, 0.80 to 1.64). The decreased risk of VTE with rivaroxaban was consistent across different doses of dabigatran (150 mg vs. 220 mg), different dosing regimens of enoxaparin in the control groups (30 mg twice daily vs. 40 mg once daily), and the type of surgery (THR vs. TKR).

SUMMARY AND DISCUSSION

We identified six good-quality SRs that evaluated thromboprophylaxis using newer oral anticoagulants versus LMWH. One SR evaluated additional drug classes, including unfractionated heparin, aspirin, and vitamin K antagonists. Although we identified no direct comparisons of newer oral anticoagulants, two good-quality SRs indirectly compared one newer oral anticoagulant with another through common comparison to enoxaparin.[21,23] Only one SR compared combined pharmacologic and mechanical thromboprophylaxis to either method alone.[9] FXa inhibitors have been studied more extensively than DTIs. In the absence of head-to-head comparisons between newer oral anticoagulants, it is difficult to draw strong conclusions on inter- or intra-drug class differences. The main findings and strength of evidence from our literature synthesis are summarized by key question in the section that follows.

SUMMARY OF EVIDENCE BY KEY QUESTION

KQ 1: Newer Oral Anticoagulants Versus Standard Treatments

FXa inhibitors. Rivaroxaban and apixaban are the most commonly studied FXa inhibitors. The risk of symptomatic DVT was reduced with FXa inhibitors thromboprophylaxis compared with LMWH, while the risk of nonfatal PE and mortality was not significantly different (all high strength of evidence). The estimated absolute risk difference was 4 fewer symptomatic DVT events for each 1000 patients receiving thromboprophylaxis with FXa inhibitors over 5 weeks compared with LMWH. However, these benefits were offset by an increase in major bleeding (moderate strength of evidence). The absolute risk difference was 2 more major bleeding events per 1000 patients on FXa thromboprophylaxis over a period of 5 weeks. Higher doses of FXa inhibitors but not intermediate or low doses were associated with increased major bleeding.[20] Subgroup analysis by specific drug and type of surgery showed a reduced risk of bleeding with apixaban compared with LMWH in TKR but not in THR; risk of major bleeding with rivaroxaban did not differ significantly for either surgery.[35] No reviews identified trials comparing oral FXa inhibitors with warfarin, UFH, or oral antiplatelet agents.

Direct thrombin inhibitors. Dabigatran is the only FDA-approved oral DTI, and the only DTI evaluated in existing SRs. Compared with LMWH, dabigatran was not associated with significant differences for any outcome examined. The strength of evidence was low for most outcomes due to few events and imprecise estimates of effect; also, effects on mortality varied substantially across studies. In addition to the major outcomes, a subgroup analysis in one SR found no significant difference between both treatment groups on bleeding requiring rehospitalization.[9] No reviews identified trials comparing oral DTIs with warfarin, unfractionated heparin, or oral antiplatelet agents.

Table 7 summarizes the findings and strength of evidence for the effects of newer oral anticoagulant drug classes compared with enoxaparin in patients undergoing THR or TKR surgery.

Table 7. Summary of the strength of evidence for KQ 1

Outcome	Number of Studies (Subjects)	Domains Pertaining to SOE				Effect Estimate (95% CI)	SOE
		Study Design/ Quality	Consistency Directness	Precision Publication Bias			
FXa vs. LMWH[a]							
Mortality (up to 10 weeks)	11 (22,838)	RCT/Good	Consistent Direct	Precise None detected		OR=0.95 (0.55 to 1.63) RD=0 (2 fewer to 1 more) deaths/1000 patients	High
Symptomatic DVT (up to 5 weeks)	18 (22,877)	RCT/Good	Consistent Direct	Precise None detected		OR=0.46 (0.30 to 0.70) RD=4 fewer (3 to 6 fewer) events/1000 patients	High
Nonfatal PE (up to 5 weeks)	20 (26,998)	RCT/Good	Consistent Direct	Precise None detected		OR=1.07 (0.65 to 1.73) RD=0 (1 fewer to 2 more) events/1000 patients	High
Major bleeding (up to 5 weeks)	21 (31,424)	RCT/Good	Inconsistent Direct	Precise None detected		OR=1.27 (0.98 to 1.65) RD=2 more (0 to 4 more) events/1000 patients	Moderate
LMWH vs. DTI[b]							
Mortality (up to 13 weeks)	4 (10,080)	RCT/Good	Inconsistent Direct	Imprecise None detected		TKR RR=1.06 (0.36 to 3.12) RD=0 (2 fewer to 6 more) events/1000 patients THR RR=1.17 (0.04 to 36.52) RD=0 (3 fewer to 107 more) events/1000 patients	Low
Symptomatic DVT (up to 5 weeks)	4 (10,264)	RCT/Good	Consistent Direct	Imprecise None detected		RR=0.82 (0.17 to 3.99) RD=2 fewer (7 fewer to 27 more) events/1000 patients	Low
Symptomatic PE (up to 5 weeks)	4 (10,264)	RCT/Good	Consistent Direct	Imprecise None detected		OR=0.69 (0.31 to 1.54) RD=1 fewer (2 fewer to 2 more) events/1000 patients	Low
Major bleeding (up to 5 weeks)	4 (10,264)	RCT/Good	Consistent Direct	Imprecise None detected		RR=0.94 (0.58 to 1.52) RD=0 (3 fewer to 3 more) events/1000 patients	Moderate
FXa or DTI vs. other antithrombotics							
All outcomes	0	NA	NA	NA		Not estimable	Insufficient

[a] Data from Neumann, 2012.
[b] Risk ratio data from Ringerike, 2012, and Gómez-Outes, 2012; risk difference calculated; SOE ratings from Sobieraj, 2012.
Notes: Outcomes are short-term; there may be some differences for hip versus knee replacement (different baseline risk and different duration of anticoagulation in existing studies); there is some evidence that FXa inhibitors at higher doses increase risk of bleeding.
Abbreviations: CI=confidence interval; DVT=deep vein thrombosis; DTI=direct thrombin inhibitor; FXa=factor X inhibitor; LMWH=low molecular weight heparin; NA=not applicable; OR=odds ratio; PE=pulmonary embolism; RCT=randomized controlled trial; RD=risk difference; RR=risk ratio; SOE=strength of evidence; THR=total hip replacement; TKR=total knee replacement

KQ 2: Combined Pharmacological and Mechanical Prophylaxis

No reviews identified trials comparing newer oral anticoagulants combined with mechanical prophylaxis to pharmacological prophylaxis alone. Even when considering standard treatments, very little data are available comparing combined-modality thromboprophylaxis and pharmacologic prophylaxis only. One SR found moderate strength of evidence that combined-modality thromboprophylaxis was associated with a decreased risk of overall DVT (including asymptomatic events) compared with pharmacologic prophylaxis only.[9] The evidence was insufficient for all other outcomes.

KQ 3: Comparisons of Individual Newer Oral Anticoagulants

Only indirect comparisons of rivaroxaban, apixaban, and dabigatran were performed through common comparison with LMWH.[23,35] These comparisons were made for only two of our major outcomes—symptomatic VTE (DVT or PE) and major bleeding. There were no significant differences in treatment effect for symptomatic VTE or major bleeding. Because these indirect comparisons are subject to confounding and the treatment effects were imprecise, we considered the strength of evidence low. Other outcomes reported included clinically relevant bleeding and net clinical endpoints. Rivaroxaban was found to be associated with an increased risk of clinically relevant bleeding, but there was no significant difference in net clinical endpoints (symptomatic VTE, major bleeding and death). Table 8 summarizes the findings and strength of evidence for between-drug comparisons of newer oral anticoagulants in patients undergoing THR or TKR.

Table 8. Summary of the strength of evidence for KQ 3

Outcome	Number of Studies (Subjects)[a]	Domains Pertaining to SOE			Effect Estimate (95% CI)	SOE
		Study Design/ Quality	Consistency Directness	Precision Publication Bias		
Apixaban, rivaroxaban, dabigatran[a]						
Mortality	NR	NA	NA	NA	Outcome not reported	Insufficient
Symptomatic DVT	NR	NA	NA	NA	Outcome not reported	Insufficient
Nonfatal PE	NR	NA	NA	NA	Outcome not reported	Insufficient
Symptomatic VTE	16 (38,747)	RCT/Good	NA Indirect	Imprecise None detected	Rivaroxaban vs. dabigatran RR=0.68 (0.21 to 2.23); RD=3 fewer (11 fewer to 4 more) events/1000 patients	Low
					Rivaroxaban vs. apixaban RR=0.59 (0.26 to 1.33) RD=4 fewer (9 fewer to 1 more)/1000 patients	Low
					Apixaban vs. dabigatran RR=1.16 (0.31 to 4.28) RD=1 more (7 fewer to 8 more)/1000 patients	Low
Major bleeding	16 (38,747)	RCT/Good	NA Indirect	Imprecise None detected	Rivaroxaban vs. dabigatran RR=1.37 (0.21 to 2.23); RD=4 more (2 fewer to 11 more) events/1000 patients	Low
					Rivaroxaban vs. apixaban RR=1.59 (0.84 to 3.02); RD=5 more (2 fewer to 12 more)/1000 patients	Low
					Apixaban vs. dabigatran RR=1.16 (0.31 to 4.28); RD=0 (8 fewer to 7 more)/1000 patients	Low

[a]Data from Gómez-Outes, 2012.
Abbreviations: DVT=deep vein thrombosis; NA=not applicable; NR=not reported; PE=pulmonary embolism; RD=risk difference; RR=risk ratio; SOE=strength of evidence; VTE=venous thromboembolism

CLINICAL AND POLICY IMPLICATIONS

Patients undergoing total knee replacement or total hip replacement are at a significant risk for VTE. The precise risk for VTE in contemporary orthopedic surgery is difficult to estimate because of changes in surgical management, the paucity of recent trials comparing thromboprophylaxis to placebo, and the high frequency of thromboprophylaxis in routine practice, making observational studies of natural history difficult to conduct. A recent, careful analysis estimated the prevalence of symptomatic VTE without thromboprophylaxis at 2.8 percent for the initial 14 days and 4.3 percent at 35 days following major orthopedic surgery.[1] Appropriate use of perioperative thromboprophylaxis significantly reduces the risk of postoperative proximal VTE, but the evidence is much more limited for effects on symptomatic DVT, PE, and mortality.[1,9]

Our evidence synthesis primarily addresses the comparative effectiveness of newer oral anticoagulants compared with standard antithrombotic agents for VTE prophylaxis. These newer drugs have been compared only to LMWH and show similar effects on most major clinical outcomes, although the strength of evidence varies by drug class and specific drug. In evaluating whether to add these newer agents to the VA formulary and whether to promote a specific thromboprophylaxis strategy, consideration should be given to the evidence of effectiveness and the importance and variability of patient values and preferences, costs, and health care system resources for successfully implementing competing strategies. In the following section, we summarize recommendations from the two major U.S. clinical guideline panels that have addressed this issue.

Guidelines

Both the American College of Chest Physicians (ACCP) and the American Academy of Orthopaedic Surgeons (AAOS) have recently issued guidelines on thromboprophylaxis in patients undergoing TKR or THR.[1,2,24] The ACCP recommends antithrombotic prophylaxis over no prophylaxis for patients undergoing TKR or THR. The AAOS guidelines suggest individual assessment of patients for thromboprophylaxis. For patients at average risk, the guidelines do not include a recommendation for a specific thromboprophylactic strategy, considering the evidence for comparative effectiveness to be inconclusive. In contrast, the ACCP guidelines make recommendations for specific strategies and include the following options: LMWH, fondaparinux, apixaban, dabigatran, rivaroxaban, low-dose unfractionated heparin, adjusted-dose vitamin K antagonists, aspirin, or an intermittent pneumatic compression device. However, in the absence of elevated bleeding risk, LMWH is recommended in preference to other agents. Factors identified as increasing the risk of bleeding include previous major bleeding, severe renal failure, concomitant antiplatelet use, and a history of or difficult-to-control surgical bleeding during the current operative procedure, extensive surgical dissection, and revision surgery.[1] For patients with increased bleeding risk, ACCP recommends intermittent pneumatic compression device or no prophylaxis.

In making recommendations, both guideline panels considered benefits and potential harms but had different approaches to considering costs. The AAOS did not conduct cost analyses and instructed guideline members to consider costs only when the impact was likely to be substantial. The ACCP process considered costs when it was plausible that resource use might change the direction or strength of recommendation and when high-quality economic analyses were available; it is not stated whether costs were considered in the recommendations pertaining to major orthopedic surgery. Guideline recommendations regarding choice of thromboprophylaxis are summarized in Table 9. Finally, we note that these guidelines address other clinical management issues, including duration and timing of thromboprophylaxis and use of routine DVT screening, which are not summarized here since they are not directly germane to our key questions.

Table 9. U.S. guideline recommendations related to specific thromboprophylaxis strategies

ACCP 2012[a]	AAOS 2011[b]
In patients undergoing THR or TKR, we recommend use of one of the following for minimum of 10–14 days rather than no antithrombotic prophylaxis: LMWH, fondaparinux, apixaban, dabigatran, rivaroxaban low-dose unfractionated heparin (LDUH), adjusted-dose VKA, aspirin (all Grade 1B) or an intermittent pneumatic compression device (IPCD) (Grade 1C).	We suggest the use of pharmacologic agents and/or mechanical compressive devices for the prevention of VTE in patients undergoing elective hip or knee arthroplasty, and who are not at elevated risk beyond that of the surgery itself for venous thromboembolism or bleeding. Grade: Moderate
In patients undergoing THR or TKR, irrespective of the concomitant use of an IPCD or length of treatment, we suggest the use of LMWH in preference to the other agents we have recommended as alternatives: fondaparinux, apixaban, dabigatran, rivaroxaban low-dose unfractionated heparin (LDUH) (all Grade 1B), adjusted-dose VKA, aspirin (all Grade 2C).	Current evidence is unclear about which prophylactic strategy is optimal or suboptimal. Therefore, we are unable to recommend for or against specific prophylactics in these patients. Grade: Inconclusive
In patients undergoing major orthopedic surgery, we suggest using dual prophylaxis with an antithrombotic agent and an IPCD during the hospital stay (Grade 2C).	In the absence of reliable evidence, patients who have had a previous VTE should receive pharmacologic prophylaxis and mechanical compressive devices. Grade: Consensus
In patients undergoing major orthopedic surgery and increased risk of bleeding, we suggest using an IPCD or no prophylaxis rather than pharmacologic treatment (Grade 2C).	In the absence of reliable evidence, patients with a known bleeding disorder and/or active liver disease should use mechanical compressive devices for preventing VTE. Grade: Consensus
In patients undergoing major orthopedic surgery and who decline or are uncooperative with injections or an IPCD, we recommend using apixaban or dabigatran (alternatively, rivaroxaban or adjusted-dose VKA if apixaban or dabigatran are unavailable) rather than other forms of prophylaxis (Grade 1B).	In the absence of reliable evidence about how long to employ these prophylactic strategies, it is the opinion of this work group that patients discuss the duration of prophylaxis with their treating physicians. Grade: Consensus

[a]ACCP evidence grading of evidence was as follows: grade 1 recommendations are strong and indicate that the benefits do or do not outweigh risks, burden, and costs, while grade 2 suggestions imply that individual patient values may lead to different choices. Furthermore, level A indicates consistent results from RCTs or observational studies with very strong association and secure generalization (high), B indicates inconsistent results from RCTs or RCTs with methodological limitations (moderate), C indicates unbiased observational studies (low), and D indicates other observational studies (e.g. case series) (very low).
[b]AAOS grading was as follows: strong when good-quality evidence, moderate when fair-quality evidence, weak when poor-quality evidence, inconclusive when insufficient or conflicting evidence, or consensus in the absence of reliable evidence.
Abbreviations: IPCD=intermittent pneumatic compression device; LDUH=low-dose unfractionated heparin; LMWH=low molecular weight heparin; THR=total hip replacement; TKR=total knee replacement; VKA=vitamin K antagonist; VTE=venous thromboembolism

APPLICABILITY

We think these results are likely to apply to Veteran populations, but recommend some caution when applying trial data to standard clinical practice. There were strict exclusion criteria for patients enrolled in these studies, including severe renal or hepatic impairment or high risk of bleeding. Patients enrolled in trials are often more adherent to treatment plans and are monitored more closely than patients in routine clinical care. As a result, treatment effects in standard clinical practice may differ from those observed in clinical trials. Furthermore, the definition of bleeding was not consistent across studies, and it did not always include surgical site bleeding, which can lead to infection, dehiscence, and reoperation. Another limitation is the treatments compared. Newer anticoagulants were compared exclusively with LMWH, an appropriate and widely used comparator, but there were no direct comparisons to other treatment options recommended by guideline panels. Finally, none of these studies included patients from the VA health care system. Compared to patients with private sector insurance, VA patients on average have a greater burden of chronic disease, which would likely increase bleeding risk. If the comparative treatment effects vary by the presence of certain comorbid conditions, these results may not be reproducible in VA settings.

STRENGTHS AND LIMITATIONS

Our study has a number of strengths, including a protocol-driven review, a comprehensive search, and careful quality assessment. Another strength is the opportunity for meta-synthesis from existing systematic reviews and the opportunity to carefully evaluate reasons for different findings or conclusions across published reviews. Limitations include the lack of head-to-head comparisons of the newer oral anticoagulants, which precludes strong conclusions on their comparative effectiveness. Further, the length of experience with these new anticoagulants is too short to allow identification of longer term adverse events that may only emerge with more widespread use.

RECOMMENDATIONS FOR FUTURE RESEARCH

We used the framework recommended by Robinson et al.[42] to identify gaps in evidence and classify why these gaps exist (Table 10).

This approach considers PICOTS (population, intervention, comparator, outcomes, timing, and setting) to identify gaps and classifies them as due to: (1) insufficient or imprecise information, (2) biased information, (3) inconsistency or unknown consistency, and (4) not the right information. VA and other health care systems should consider their clinical and policy needs when deciding whether to invest in research to address gaps in evidence. Specific research questions can be evaluated quantitatively, using value-of-information analysis, which uses Bayesian methods to estimate the potential benefits of gathering further information through research.[43]

Table 10. Evidence gaps and future research

Evidence Gap	Reason	Type of Studies to Consider
Absence of direct comparisons between newer anticoagulant drugs	Insufficient information	Multicenter RCTs High-quality network meta-analyses Observational comparative effectiveness studies
Absence of direct comparisons between newer anticoagulants and agents other than LMWH	Insufficient information	Multicenter RCTs Observational comparative effectiveness studies
Absence of comparisons between combined treatment with newer anticoagulants and mechanical thromboprophylaxis to pharmacological thromboprophylaxis alone	Insufficient information	Multicenter RCTs Observational comparative effectiveness studies
Adverse effects with long-term use and in usual clinical practice	Insufficient information	Observational studies

Abbreviations: LMWH=low molecular weight heparin; RCT=randomized controlled trial

CONCLUSION

For THR or TKR, the 35-day rate of symptomatic VTE without thromboprophylaxis is estimated to be 4.3 percent. Pharmacological thromboprophylaxis decreases VTE by approximately 50 percent but with the tradeoff of increased bleeding. Newer oral anticoagulants have a more convenient route of administration compared with LMWH, and unlike adjusted dose warfarin, they do not require regular laboratory monitoring. Compared with LMWH, FXa inhibitors are associated with a reduced risk of symptomatic DVT, but mortality and nonfatal PE are not significantly different, and the risk of major bleeding episodes is increased.

There are no available studies on head-to-head comparisons of these novel anticoagulants. Longer clinical experience and direct drug-drug comparisons are needed to better assess the risk-to-benefit ratio of newer oral anticoagulants for surgical thromboprophylaxis. Based on current evidence, newer anticoagulants—particularly FXa inhibitors—are a reasonable option for thromboprophylaxis in patients undergoing total hip replacement or total knee replacement.

REFERENCES

1. Falck-Ytter Y, Francis CW, Johanson NA, et al. Prevention of VTE in orthopedic surgery patients: Antithrombotic Therapy and Prevention of Thrombosis, 9th ed: American College of Chest Physicians Evidence-Based Clinical Practice Guidelines. *Chest.* 2012;141(2 Suppl):e278S-325S.

2. Mont MA, Jacobs JJ, Boggio LN, et al. Preventing venous thromboembolic disease in patients undergoing elective hip and knee arthroplasty. *J Am Acad Orthop Surg.* 2011;19(12):768-76.

3. Hill J, Treasure T. Reducing the risk of venous thromboembolism (deep vein thrombosis and pulmonary embolism) in inpatients having surgery: summary of NICE guidance. *BMJ.* 2007;334(7602):1053-4.

4. Friedman RJ, Gallus A, Gil-Garay E, et al. Practice patterns in the use of venous thromboembolism prophylaxis after total joint arthroplasty—insights from the Multinational Global Orthopaedic Registry (GLORY). *Am J Orthop (Belle Mead NJ).* 2010;39(9 Suppl):14-21.

5. Binns M, Pho R. Femoral vein occlusion during hip arthroplasty. *Clin Orthop Relat Res.* 1990(255):168-72.

6. Clark C, Cotton LT. Blood-flow in deep veins of leg. Recording technique and evaluation of methods to increase flow during operation. *Br J Surg.* 1968;55(3):211-4.

7. Planes A, Vochelle N, Fagola M. Total hip replacement and deep vein thrombosis. A venographic and necropsy study. *J Bone Joint Surg Br.* 1990;72(1):9-13.

8. Sharrock NE, Go G, Harpel PC, et al. The John Charnley Award. Thrombogenesis during total hip arthroplasty. *Clin Orthop Relat Res.* 1995(319):16-27.

9. Sobieraj DM, Coleman CI, Tongbram V, et al. Venous Thromboembolism in Orthopedic Surgery. Comparative Effectiveness Review No. 49. (Prepared by the University of Connecticut/Hartford Hospital Evidence-based Practice Center under Contract No. 290-2007-10067-I.) AHRQ Publication No. 12-EHC020-EF. Rockville, MD: Agency for Healthcare Research and Quality. March 2012.Available at: www.effectivehealthcare.ahrq.gov/reports/final.cfm. Accessed November 7, 2012.

10. Lieberman JR, Hsu WK. Prevention of venous thromboembolic disease after total hip and knee arthroplasty. *J Bone Joint Surg Am.* 2005;87(9):2097-112.

11. Molnar RB, Jenkin DE, Millar MJ, et al. The Australian arthroplasty thromboprophylaxis survey. *J Arthroplasty.* 2012;27(2):173-9.

12. Ettema HB, Mulder MC, Nurmohamed MT, et al. Dutch orthopedic thromboprophylaxis: a 5-year follow-up survey. *Acta Orthop.* 2009;80(1):109-12.

13. Hirsh J, Levine MN. Low molecular weight heparin: laboratory properties and clinical evaluation. A review. *Eur J Surg Suppl.* 1994(571):9-22.

14. Weitz JI. Low-molecular-weight heparins. *N Engl J Med.* 1997;337(10):688-98.

15. Turpie AG. Pentasaccharide Org31540/SR90107A clinical trials update: lessons for practice. *Am Heart J.* 2001;142(2 Suppl):S9-15.

16. Fareed J, Thethi I, Hoppensteadt D. Old versus new oral anticoagulants: focus on pharmacology. *Annu Rev Pharmacol Toxicol.* 2012;52:79-99.

17. Moher D, Liberati A, Tetzlaff J, et al. Preferred reporting items for systematic reviews and meta-analyses: the PRISMA statement. *J Clin Epidemiol.* 2009;62(10):1006-12.

18. Montori VM, Wilczynski NL, Morgan D, et al. Optimal search strategies for retrieving systematic reviews from MEDLINE: analytical survey. *BMJ.* 2005;330(7482):68.

19. Shojania KG, Bero LA. Taking advantage of the explosion of systematic reviews: an efficient MEDLINE search strategy. *Eff Clin Pract.* 2001;4(4):157-62.

20. Neumann I, Rada G, Claro JC, et al. Oral direct factor Xa inhibitors versus low-molecular-weight heparin to prevent venous thromboembolism in patients undergoing total hip or knee replacement a systematic review and meta-analysis. *Ann Intern Med.* 2012;156(10):710-719.

21. Loke YK, Kwok CS. Dabigatran and rivaroxaban for prevention of venous thromboembolism--systematic review and adjusted indirect comparison. *J Clin Pharm Ther.* 2011;36(1):111-24.

22. Ringerike T, Hamidi V, Hagen G, et al. Thromboprophylactic treatment with rivaroxaban or dabigatran compared with enoxaparin or dalteparin in patients undergoing elective hip- or knee replacement surgery. Report from NOKC nr 13 - 2011. *Health Technology Assessment (HTA).* 2011.

23. Gómez-Outes A, Terleira-Fernández AI, Suárez-Gea ML, et al. Dabigatran, rivaroxaban, or apixaban versus enoxaparin for thromboprophylaxis after total hip or knee replacement: systematic review, meta-analysis, and indirect treatment comparisons. *BMJ.* 2012;344.

24. Jacobs JJ, Mont MA, Bozic KJ, et al. American Academy of Orthopaedic Surgeons clinical practice guideline on: preventing venous thromboembolic disease in patients undergoing elective hip and knee arthroplasty. *J Bone Joint Surg Am.* 2012;94(8):746-7.

25. Marinopoulos SS, Dorman T, Ratanawongsa N, et al. Effectiveness of continuing medical education. *Evid Rep Technol Assess (Full Rep).* 2007(149):1-69.

26. Moher D, Cook DJ, Eastwood S, et al. Improving the quality of reports of meta-analyses of randomised controlled trials: the QUOROM statement. Quality of Reporting of Meta-analyses. *Lancet.* 1999;354(9193):1896-900.

27. Shea BJ, Grimshaw JM, Wells GA, et al. Development of AMSTAR: a measurement tool to assess the methodological quality of systematic reviews. *BMC Med Res Methodol.* 2007;7:10.

28. Mills EJ, Ioannidis JP, Thorlund K, et al. How to use an article reporting a multiple treatment comparison meta-analysis. *JAMA*. 2012;308(12):1246-53.

29. Agency for Healthcare Research and Quality. Methods Guide for Effectiveness and Comparative Effectiveness Reviews. Rockville, MD: Agency for Healthcare Research and Quality. Available at: www.effectivehealthcare.ahrq.gov/search-for-guides-reviews-and-reports/?pageaction=displayproduct&mp=1&productID=318. Accessed August 1, 2012.

30. Guyatt GH, Oxman AD, Kunz R, et al. GRADE guidelines 6. Rating the quality of evidence--imprecision. *J Clin Epidemiol*. 2011;64(12):1283-93.

31. Schunemann HJ, Oxman AD, Brozek J, et al. Grading quality of evidence and strength of recommendations for diagnostic tests and strategies. *BMJ*. 2008;336(7653):1106-10.

32. Cao YB, Zhang JD, Shen H, et al. Rivaroxaban versus enoxaparin for thromboprophylaxis after total hip or knee arthroplasty: a meta-analysis of randomized controlled trials. *Eur J Clin Pharmacol*. 2010;66(11):1099-108.

33. Huang J, Cao Y, Liao C, et al. Apixaban versus enoxaparin in patients with total knee arthroplasty. A meta-analysis of randomised trials. *Thromb Haemost*. 2011;105(2):245-53.

34. Turun S, Banghua L, Yuan Y, et al. A systematic review of rivaroxaban versus enoxaparin in the prevention of venous thromboembolism after hip or knee replacement. *Thromb Res*. 2011;127(6):525-34.

35. Alves C, Batel-Marques F, Macedo AF. Apixaban and Rivaroxaban Safety After Hip and Knee Arthroplasty: A Meta-Analysis. *J Cardiovasc Pharmacol Ther*. 2011.

36. Eriksson BI, Borris LC, Friedman RJ, et al. Rivaroxaban versus enoxaparin for thromboprophylaxis after hip arthroplasty. *N Engl J Med*. 2008;358(26):2765-75.

37. Kakkar AK, Brenner B, Dahl OE, et al. Extended duration rivaroxaban versus short-term enoxaparin for the prevention of venous thromboembolism after total hip arthroplasty: a double-blind, randomised controlled trial. *Lancet*. 2008;372(9632):31-9.

38. Lassen MR, Ageno W, Borris LC, et al. Rivaroxaban versus enoxaparin for thromboprophylaxis after total knee arthroplasty. *N Engl J Med*. 2008;358(26):2776-86.

39. Turpie AG, Lassen MR, Davidson BL, et al. Rivaroxaban versus enoxaparin for thromboprophylaxis after total knee arthroplasty (RECORD4): a randomised trial. *Lancet*. 2009;373(9676):1673-80.

40. Eriksson BI, Dahl OE, Buller HR, et al. A new oral direct thrombin inhibitor, dabigatran etexilate, compared with enoxaparin for prevention of thromboembolic events following total hip or knee replacement: the BISTRO II randomized trial. *J Thromb Haemost*. 2005;3(1):103-11.

41. Bucher HC, Guyatt GH, Griffith LE, et al. The results of direct and indirect treatment comparisons in meta-analysis of randomized controlled trials. *J Clin Epidemiol*. 1997;50(6):683-91.

42. Robinson KA, Saldanha IJ, Mckoy NA. Frameworks for Determining Research Gaps During Systematic Reviews. Methods Future Research Needs Report No. 2. (Prepared by the Johns Hopkins University Evidence-based Practice Center under Contract No. HHSA 290-2007-10061-I.) AHRQ Publication No. 11-EHC043-EF. Rockville, MD: Agency for Healthcare Research and Quality. June 2011. Available at: www.effectivehealthcare.ahrq.gov/reports/final.cfm. Accessed May 22, 2012.

43. Myers E, McBroom AJ, Shen L, et al. Value-of-Information Analysis for Patient-Centered Outcomes Research Prioritization. Report prepared by the Duke Evidence-based Practice Center. Patient-Centered Outcomes Research Institute. March 2012.

APPENDIX A. SEARCH STRATEGIES

Table A-1. Search strategy for PubMed (5/29/2012, updated 9/28/2012)

Set #	Terms	Results
1	Dabigatran[tiab] OR desirudin[tiab] OR edoxaban[tiab] OR rivaroxaban[tiab] OR apixaban[tiab] OR betrixaban[tiab] OR YM150[tiab] OR razaxaban[tiab] OR "dabigatran etexilate"[Supplementary Concept] OR "desirudin"[Supplementary Concept] OR "edoxaban"[Supplementary Concept] OR "rivaroxaban"[Supplementary Concept] OR "apixaban"[Supplementary Concept] OR "betrixaban"[Supplementary Concept] OR "razaxaban hydrochloride"[Supplementary Concept] OR "factor Xa, Glu-Gly-Arg-"[Supplementary Concept] OR "KFA1411"[Supplementary Concept]	1319
2	(((knee[tiab] OR hip[tiab] OR elbow[ti]) AND (replacement[tiab] OR Arthroplasty[tiab]))) OR ("Orthopedic Procedures"[Mesh])	194066
3	#1 AND #2	298
4	("Review"[Publication Type] OR "Review Literature as Topic"[Mesh]) OR ("Meta-Analysis as Topic"[Mesh] OR "Meta-Analysis"[Publication Type]) OR systematic[sb]	1782948
5	#3 AND #4	117

Table A-2. Search strategy for Embase (5/30/2012, updated 9/28/2012)

Set #	Terms	Results
1	'dabigatran'/exp OR dabigatran OR 'desirudin'/exp OR desirudin OR 'edoxaban'/exp OR edoxaban OR 'rivaroxaban'/exp OR rivaroxaban OR 'apixaban'/exp OR apixaban OR'betrixaban'/exp OR betrixaban OR 'ym150'/exp OR ym150 OR 'razaxaban'/exp OR razaxaban OR 'factor xa inhibitors' OR 'factor xa inhibitor'/exp OR 'factor xa inhibitor' OR 'fxa inhibitors' OR 'fxa inhibitor' OR'direct thrombin inhibitor' OR 'direct thrombin inhibitors' OR dtis OR 'novel anticoagulants' OR 'new anticoagulants' OR 'novel anticoagulant' OR 'new anticoagulant'	10942
2	'orthopedic surgery'/exp OR (hip:ab,ti OR knee:ab,ti OR elbow:ab,ti AND (replacement:ab,ti OR arthroplasty:ab,ti))	351,364
3	#1 AND #2	1522
4	#3 limited to Systematic reviews or meta –analysis AND (embase)/lim NOT (medline)/lim	43

Table A-3. Search strategy for Cochrane Database of Systematic Reviews (5/30/2012, updated 9/28/2012)

Set #	Term	Results
1	dabigatran OR desirudin OR edoxaban OR rivaroxaban OR apixaban OR betrixaban OR YM150 OR razaxaban OR "factor Xa inhibitors" OR "factor Xa inhibitor" OR "fxa inhibitors" OR "fxa inhibitor" OR "direct thrombin inhibitor" OR "direct thrombin inhibitors" OR DTIs OR "novel anticoagulants" OR "new anticoagulants" OR "novel anticoagulant" OR "new anticoagulant"	472
2	MeSH descriptor Orthopedic Procedures explode all trees OR (knee):ti,ab,kw or (elbow):ti,ab,kw AND (replacement):ti,ab,kw or (arthroplasty):ti,ab,kw	8138
3	#1 AND #2	117
4	#3 limited to Systematic reviews or meta-analysis	8

APPENDIX B. EXCLUDED STUDIES

All citations listed in Table B-1 were reviewed in their full-text version and excluded for the reason indicated. An alphabetical reference list follows the table.

Table B-1. Excluded studies with reasons

Reference	Not a systematic review	Does not address Key Questions
Cohen, 2012	X[a]	
Dahl, 2009	X	
Dahl, 2010	X	
Diamantopoulos, 2010	X	
Duggan, 2009	X	
Eriksson, 2011	X	
Eriksson, 2009	X	
Falck-Ytter, 2012	X	
Friedman, 2011	X	
Friedman, 2010	X	
Friedman, 2011	X	
Goff, 2011	X	
Gomez-Outes, 2011	X	
Gras, 2011	X	
Holmes, 2009	X	
Hull, 2010	X	
Imberti, 2009	X	
Jacobs, 2012	X	
Kwong, 2011	X	
Kwong, 2011	X	
Lazo-Langner, 2009	X	
Lee, 2012	X	
Lereun, 2011	X	
Mantha, 2011	X	
Maratea, 2011	X	
Melillo, 2010		X
Merli, 2009	X	
Miller, 2012		X
Mont, 2011	X	
Nieto, 2012	X	
Poultsides, 2012		X
Prom, 2011		X
Raskob, 2012	X	
Stevenson, 2009	X	
Trkulja, 2010	X	
Watkins, 2011	X	
Wolowacz, 2011		X
Wolowacz, 2009	X	

[a]Rated as poor-quality systematic review and excluded.

LIST OF EXCLUDED STUDIES

Cohen A, Drost P, Marchant N, et al. The efficacy and safety of pharmacological prophylaxis of venous thromboembolism following elective knee or hip replacement: systematic review and network meta-analysis. *Clin Appl Thromb Hemost.* 2012;18(6):611-627.

Dahl OE. Dabigatran etexilate for the prophylaxis of venous thromboembolism after hip or knee replacement rationale for dose regimen. *Clin Appl Thromb Hemost.* 2009;15 Suppl 1:17S-24S.

Dahl OE, Quinlan DJ, Bergqvist D, et al. A critical appraisal of bleeding events reported in venous thromboembolism prevention trials of patients undergoing hip and knee arthroplasty. *J Thromb Haemost.* 2010;8(9):1966-75.

Diamantopoulos A, Lees M, Wells PS, et al. Cost-effectiveness of rivaroxaban versus enoxaparin for the prevention of postsurgical venous thromboembolism in Canada. *Thromb Haemost.* 2010;104(4):760-70.

Duggan ST, Scott LJ, Plosker GL. Rivaroxaban: a review of its use for the prevention of venous thromboembolism after total hip or knee replacement surgery. *Drugs.* 2009;69(13):1829-51.

Eriksson BI, Dahl OE, Huo MH, et al. Oral dabigatran versus enoxaparin for thromboprophylaxis after primary total hip arthroplasty (RE-NOVATE II*). A randomised, double-blind, non-inferiority trial. *Thromb Haemost.* 2011;105(4):721-9.

Eriksson BI, Friedman RJ. Dabigatran etexilate: pivotal trials for venous thromboembolism prophylaxis after hip or knee arthroplasty. *Clin Appl Thromb Hemost.* 2009;15 Suppl 1:25S-31S.

Falck-Ytter Y, Francis CW, Johanson NA, et al. Prevention of VTE in orthopedic surgery patients: Antithrombotic Therapy and Prevention of Thrombosis, 9th ed: American College of Chest Physicians Evidence-Based Clinical Practice Guidelines. *Chest.* 2012;141(2 Suppl):e278S-325S.

Friedman RJ. Novel oral anticoagulants for VTE prevention in orthopedic surgery: overview of phase 3 trials. *Orthopedics.* 2011;34(10):795-804.

Friedman RJ, Dahl OE, Rosencher N, et al. Dabigatran versus enoxaparin for prevention of venous thromboembolism after hip or knee arthroplasty: a pooled analysis of three trials. *Thromb Res.* 2010;126(3):175-82.

Friedman RJ, Sengupta N, Lees M. Economic impact of venous thromboembolism after hip and knee arthroplasty: potential impact of rivaroxaban. *Expert Rev Pharmacoecon Outcomes Res.* 2011;11(3):299-306.

Goff T, Kontakis G, Giannoudis PV. Safety and efficacy of rivaroxaban for thromboprophylaxis following lower limb surgery: an update. *Expert Opin Drug Saf.* 2011;10(5):687-96.

Gomez-Outes A, Terleira-Fernandez A, Suarez-Gea ML, et al. New oral anticoagulants for thromboprophylaxis after total hip or knee replacement: A meta-analysis and indirect treatment comparisons. *Basic and Clinical Pharmacology and Toxicology.* 2011;109:34.

Gras J. Edoxaban for the prevention of thromboembolic events after surgery. *Drugs Today (Barc).* 2011;47(10):753-61.

Holmes M, Carroll C, Papaioannou D. Dabigatran etexilate for the prevention of venous thromboembolism in patients undergoing elective hip and knee surgery: a single technology appraisal. *Health Technol Assess.* 2009;13 Suppl 2:55-62.

Hull RD, Liang J, Brant R. Pooled analysis of trials may, in the presence of heterogeneity inadvertently lead to fragile conclusions due to the importance of clinically relevant variables being either hidden or lost when the findings are pooled. *Thromb Res.* 2010;126(3):164-5.

Imberti D, Dall'Asta C, Pierfranceschi MG. Oral factor Xa inhibitors for thromboprophylaxis in major orthopedic surgery: a review. *Intern Emerg Med.* 2009;4(6):471-7.

Jacobs JJ, Mont MA, Bozic KJ, et al. American Academy of Orthopaedic Surgeons clinical practice guideline on: preventing venous thromboembolic disease in patients undergoing elective hip and knee arthroplasty. J Bone Joint Surg Am. 2012;94(8):746-7.

Kwong LM. Therapeutic potential of rivaroxaban in the prevention of venous thromboembolism following hip and knee replacement surgery: a review of clinical trial data. *Vasc Health Risk Manag.* 2011;7:461-6.

Kwong LM. Cost-effectiveness of rivaroxaban after total hip or total knee arthroplasty. *Am J Manag Care.* 2011;17(1 Suppl):S22-6.

Lazo-Langner A, Hawell J, Kovacs MJ, et al. A systematic review and meta-analysis of proportions of thrombosis and bleeding in patients receiving venous thromboembolism (VTE) prophylaxis after orthopedic surgery (OS). an update. *Blood.* 2009;114(22).

Lee S, White CM. Upcoming oral factor Xa inhibitors for venous thromboembolism prophylaxis in patients undergoing major orthopedic surgery: rivaroxaban (Xarelto) and apixaban (Eliquis) review. *Conn Med.* 2012;76(1):39-42.

Lereun C, Wells P, Diamantopoulos A, et al. An indirect comparison, via enoxaparin, of rivaroxaban with dabigatran in the prevention of venous thromboembolism after hip or knee replacement. *J Med Econ.* 2011;14(2):238-44.

Mantha S. Oral factor Xa inhibitors vs. enoxaparin for thromboprophylaxis after joint replacement surgery: A meta-analysis. *Journal of Thrombosis and Haemostasis.* 2011;9:189.

Maratea D, Fadda V, Trippoli S, et al. Prevention of venous thromboembolism after major orthopedic surgery: indirect comparison of three new oral anticoagulants. *J Thromb Haemost.* 2011;9(9):1868-70.

Melillo SN, Scanlon JV, Exter BP, et al. Rivaroxaban for thromboprophylaxis in patients undergoing major orthopedic surgery. *Ann Pharmacother.* 2010;44(6):1061-71.

Merli G, Spyropoulos AC, Caprini JA. Use of emerging oral anticoagulants in clinical practice: translating results from clinical trials to orthopedic and general surgical patient populations. *Ann Surg.* 2009;250(2):219-28.

Miller CS, Grandi SM, Shimony A, et al. Meta-Analysis of Efficacy and Safety of New Oral Anticoagulants (Dabigatran, Rivaroxaban, Apixaban) Versus Warfarin in Patients With Atrial Fibrillation. *Am J Cardiol.* 2012.

Mont MA, Jacobs JJ, Boggio LN, et al. Preventing venous thromboembolic disease in patients undergoing elective hip and knee arthroplasty. *J Am Acad Orthop Surg.* 2011;19(12):768-76.

Nieto JA, Espada NG, Merino RG, et al. Dabigatran, Rivaroxaban and Apixaban versus Enoxaparin for thomboprophylaxis after total knee or hip arthroplasty: Pool-analysis of phase III randomized clinical trials. *Thromb Res.* 2012;130(2):183-91.

Poultsides LA, Gonzalez Della Valle A, Memtsoudis SG, et al. Meta-analysis of cause of death following total joint replacement using different thromboprophylaxis regimens. *J Bone Joint Surg Br.* 2012;94(1):113-21.

Prom R, Spinler SA. The role of apixaban for venous and arterial thromboembolic disease. *Ann Pharmacother.* 2011;45(10):1262-83.

Raskob GE, Gallus AS, Pineo GF, et al. Apixaban versus enoxaparin for thromboprophylaxis after hip or knee replacement: pooled analysis of major venous thromboembolism and bleeding in 8464 patients from the ADVANCE-2 and ADVANCE-3 trials. *J Bone Joint Surg Br.* 2012;94(2):257-64.

Stevenson M, Scope A, Holmes M, et al. Rivaroxaban for the prevention of venous thromboembolism: a single technology appraisal. *Health Technol Assess.* 2009;13 Suppl 3:43-8.

Trkulja V, Kolundzic R. Rivaroxaban vs dabigatran for thromboprophylaxis after joint-replacement surgery: exploratory indirect comparison based on meta-analysis of pivotal clinical trials. *Croat Med J.* 2010;51(2):113-23.

Watkins PB, Desai M, Berkowitz SD, et al. Evaluation of drug-induced serious hepatotoxicity (eDISH): application of this data organization approach to phase III clinical trials of rivaroxaban after total hip or knee replacement surgery. *Drug Saf.* 2011;34(3):243-52.

Wolowacz SE. Pharmacoeconomics of dabigatran etexilate for prevention of thromboembolism after joint replacement surgery. *Expert Rev Pharmacoecon Outcomes Res.* 2011;11(1):9-25.

Wolowacz SE, Roskell NS, Plumb JM, et al. Efficacy and safety of dabigatran etexilate for the prevention of venous thromboembolism following total hip or knee arthroplasty. A meta-analysis. *Thromb Haemost.* 2009;101(1):77-85.

APPENDIX C. SAMPLE DATA ABSTRACTION FORM

First author, year, Reference Library#

STATED OBJECTIVE OF PAPER: " "

METHODS:

Databases accessed for literature search: X, Y, Z… and abstracts of (meetings, Websites, etc.):

Search date:

Language limits for search:

Inclusion criteria: Cut and paste from article AND ensure the following are addressed:
- *Study design type:*
- *Patients*: Any characteristic that would include or exclude (e.g., under 18 years)
- *Intervention*: Drugs of interest
- *Comparator*: What is considered a valid comparator for the drug of interest?
- *Outcomes*: Any of the following (also provide any definitions given by the authors):
    1. All-cause mortality
    2. VTE-related mortality
    3. VTE (only if DVT and PE not given separately)
    4. Symptomatic DVT
    5. Nonfatal PE
    6. Serious AEs
    7. Fatal bleeding
    8. Major bleeding
    9. Bleeding from the surgical site
    10. Rehospitalization (includes bleeding that requires reoperation).

Exclusion criteria: Cut and paste from article

Summary of analysis approach:
- System used (RevMan, Peto, CMA, etc.)
- Report statistic (OR, RR, RD, MD, combination?)
- Special procedures (double-checking, etc.)
- Heterogeneity addressed?
- Publication bias addressed?
- Subgroup analyses?
- Sensitivity analyses?
-

Funding Source: Look carefully for pharma $

QUALITY: See separate quality rating form

RESULTS: Number of key questions: XX (if multiple KQs, complete this section for each KQ)

A. Number of studies included (if numbers vary by KQ, give total and number for each KQ):
XX met eligibility; XX analyzed (were any articles specific excluded, why?)

B. Patient characteristics (range across studies):
Type of surgery: Knee replacement (n=); hip replacement (n=); either knee or hip (n=)
Sex (female-n %): ---- to ---- (XX.X to XX.X%)
Sample size (n): YY to YY,YYY
Mean age (years): ZZ.Z to ZZ.Z
Mean BMI or weight: AA.A to AA.A
Veteran settings, if given:
Risk factors for bleeding (prior GI bleed, anemia, renal insufficiency, DM):
Intervention drugs: (generic name, number of studies, notes about dosage)
　　　1. KQ1 – newer oral anticoagulants (FXa or DTI)
　　　2. KQ2 – combined pharmacological (any type) + mechanical modalities
　　　3. KQ3 – new oral anticoagulant (FXa or DTI)

Comparator:
　　　1. KQ1 – LMWH, UFH, warfarin, aspirin
　　　2. KQ2 – pharmacological treatment alone
　　　3. KQ3 – other newer oral anticoagulant (FXa or DTI) – direct or indirect comparison

Concurrent other drug administration? (yes/no)
- Antiplatelet drugs:
- Other

C. Outcomes: (FXa vs LMWH)
Outcomes definition:
　　　Were they objectively evaluated?
　　　Was there missing data?
　　　Other specifics mentioned about quality of results:

Duration of anticoagulation:
- Knee: e.g., 5–14 days (n=)
　　　≥15 days (n=)
- Hip: e.g., < 28 days (n=)
　　　≥ 28 days (n=)

Followup timing:
- e.g., <14 days (n=)
- 14–30 days (n=)
- > 30 days (n=)
-

Risk of bias for primary studies: Any standard ratings given? Specific issues? (e.g., blinding? adjudication? poor completion rates?)

Quantitative summaries: Give # participants, # studies, summary estimate and 95% CI, I^2, RD (per 1,000), strength of evidence (SOE) if given. [For example: 22,838 participants, 11 studies; OR 0.95 (95% CI, 0.55 to 1.63); I^2=43%; RD=0 fewer events (CI, 2 fewer to 1 more) per 1,000; SOE=High]

Provide these data for the following outcomes, if given:
Mortality:
VTE-related mortality:
Total VTE:
Symptomatic DVT:
Nonfatal PE:
Serious AEs:
Major bleeding:
Bleeding from the surgical site:
Rehospitalization: (give reason if possible)
Other outcome of significance:

Did they measure publication bias? (via funnel plots, etc.)

Subgroup analyses: If presented, give type and outcome
    Dose:
    Type of surgery:
    Within drug class:
    Multiple treatments:

Sensitivity analysis: If presented, give type and outcome

AUTHOR'S CONCLUSION: (take-home message): " "

APPENDIX D. CRITERIA USED IN QUALITY ASSESSMENT OF SYSTEMATIC REVIEWS

For reviews, first determine whether it is a systematic review. To be a systematic review, it must include a methods section that describes (1) a search strategy and (2) an a priori approach to synthesizing the data. For reviews determined to meet the systematic review criteria, assess methodological quality.*

General instructions: The purpose of this rating tool is to evaluate the scientific quality of systematic reviews. It is not intended to measure the literary quality, importance, relevance, originality, or other attributes of systematic reviews.

Step 1: Grade each criterion listed below as "Yes," "No," "Can't tell" or "Not Applicable." Factors to consider when making an assessment are listed under each criterion. Where appropriate (particularly when assigning a "No," or "Can't tell" score), please provide a brief rationale for your decision (in parentheses).

1. **Is a focused clinical question clearly stated?**
   At a minimum, the question should be developed <u>a priori</u> and should clearly identify population and outcomes. The study question does not have to be in PICO format (Population, Intervention, Comparisons, Outcomes.)
   [] Yes   [] No   [] Can't tell   [] N/A

2. **Are the search methods used to identify relevant studies clearly described?**
   Search methods described in enough detail to permit replication (The report must include search date, databases used, and search terms (Key words and/or MESH terms must be stated and where feasible the search strategy should be provided.)
   [] Yes   [] No   [] Can't tell   [] N/A

3. **Was a comprehensive literature search performed?**
   At least 2 electronic sources should be searched and electronic searches should be supplemented by consulting: reference lists from prior reviews, textbooks, or included studies; specialized registries (e.g., Cochrane registries); or queries to experts in the field.
   [] Yes   [] No   [] Can't tell   [] N/A

4. **Was selection bias avoided?**
   Study reports the number of studies identified through searches, the numbers excluded, and gives appropriate reasons for excluding – based on explicit inclusion/exclusion criteria.
   [] Yes   [] No   [] Can't tell   [] N/A

5. **Was there duplicate study selection and data extraction?**
   Did two or more raters make inclusion/exclusion decisions, abstract data, and assess study quality – either independently or with one rater over-reading the first raters result? Was an appropriate method used to resolve disagreements (e.g., a consensus procedure)?
   [] Yes   [] No   [] Can't tell   [] N/A

6. **Were the characteristics of the included studies provided?**
   In an aggregated form such as a table, data from the original studies should be provided on the participants, interventions and outcomes. The ranges of characteristics in all the studies analyzed (e.g., age, race, sex, relevant socioeconomic data, disease status, duration, severity or other diseases) should be reported.
   [] Yes   [] No   [] Can't tell   [] N/A

7. **Was the scientific quality of the included studies assessed and documented?**
   A priori methods of assessment should be provided and criteria used to assess study quality specified in enough detail to permit replication.
   [] Yes   [] No   [] Can't tell   [] N/A

8. **Were the methods used to combine the findings of studies appropriate?**
   For pooled results, an accepted quantitative method of pooling should be used (i.e., more than simple addition; e.g., random-effects or fixed-effect model). For pooled results, a qualitative and quantitative assessment of homogeneity (Cochran's Q and/or I^2) should be performed. If only qualitative analyses are completed, the study should describe the reasons that quantitative analyses were not completed.
   [] Yes   [] No   [] Can't tell   [] N/A

9. **Was the scientific quality of the included studies used appropriately in formulating conclusions?**
   The results of the methodological rigor and scientific quality should be considered in the analysis (e.g. subgroup analyses) and the conclusions of the review, and explicitly stated in formulating recommendations.
   [] Yes   [] No   [] Can't tell   [] N/A

10. **Was publication bias assessed?**
    Publication bias tested using funnel plots, test statistics (e.g., Egger's regression test), and/or search of trials registry for unpublished studies.
    [] Yes   [] No   [] Can't tell   [] N/A

11. **Was the conflict of interest stated?**
    Potential sources of support should be clearly acknowledged in both the systematic review and the included studies.
    [] Yes   [] No   [] Can't tell   [] N/A

12. **Are the stated conclusions supported by the data presented?**
    Were the conclusions made by the author(s) supported by the data and/or analyses reported in the systematic review?
    [] Yes   [] No   [] Can't tell   [] N/A

Step 2: Rate the overall quality of the SR as "Good," "Fair," or "Poor" using the guidance below.

Good = After considering items 1-12, item 12 is rated "Yes" with no important limitations. This means that few of the items 1-12 are rated "No," and none of the limitations are thought to decrease the validity of the conclusions. If items 3, 4, 7, or 8 are rated "No," then the review is likely to have major flaws

Fair = After considering items 1-12, item 12 is rated "Yes," but with at least some important limitations. This means that enough of the items 1-12 are rated "No" to introduce some uncertainty about the validity of the conclusions.

Poor = After considering items 1-12, item 12 is rated "No." This means that several of items 1-12 are rated "No," introducing serious uncertainty about the validity of the conclusions.

*Adapted from:

1. Shea BJ, Grimshaw JM, Wells GA, et al. Development of AMSTAR: a measurement tool to assess the methodological quality of systematic reviews. BMC Med Res Methodol. 2007;7:10.

2. Moher D, Cook DJ, Eastwood S, et al. Improving the quality of reports of meta-analyses of randomised controlled trials: the QUOROM statement. Quality of Reporting of Meta-analyses. Lancet. 1999;354(9193):1896-900.

3. Marinopoulos SS, Dorman T, Ratanawongsa N, et al. Effectiveness of continuing medical education. Evid Rep Technol Assess (Full Rep). 2007(149):1-69.

Table D-1 shows the quality ratings for the systematic reviews included in this evidence report.

Table D-1. Quality assessment for included systematic reviews

Criteria for grading the quality of a systematic review (SR)	Neumann, 2012	Sobieraj, 2012	Gomez-Outes, 2012	Loke, 2011	Ringerike, 2011	Alves, 2011
Q1. Is a focused clinical question clearly stated?	Yes	Yes	Yes	Yes	Yes	Yes
Q2. Are the search methods used to identify relevant studies clearly described?	Yes	Yes	Yes	Yes	Yes	Yes
Q3. Was a comprehensive literature search performed?	Yes	Yes	Yes	Yes	Yes	Yes
Q4. Was selection bias avoided?	Yes	Yes	Yes	Yes	Yes	Yes
Q5. Was there duplicate study selection and data extraction?	Yes	Yes	Yes	Yes	Yes	Yes
Q6. Were the characteristics of the included studies provided?	Yes	Yes	Yes	Yes	No	Yes
Q7. Was the scientific quality of the included studies assessed and documented?	Yes	Yes	Yes	Yes	Yes	Can't tell
Q8. Were the methods used to combine the findings of studies appropriate?	Yes	Yes	Yes	Yes	Yes	Yes
Q9. Was the scientific quality of the included studies used appropriate in formulating conclusions?	Yes	Yes	Yes	Yes	Yes	Yes
Q10. Was publication bias assessed?	Yes	Yes	Yes	Yes	Yes	Yes
Q11. Was the conflict of interest stated?	Yes	Yes	Yes	Yes	Can't tell	Yes
Q12. Are the stated conclusions supported by the data presented?	Yes	Yes	Yes	Yes	Yes	Yes
Overall quality	Good	Good	Good	Good	Good	Good

APPENDIX E. PEER REVIEW COMMENTS

Reviewer	Comment	Response
Question 1: Are the objectives, scope, and methods for this review clearly described?		
1	Yes. Objectives are clear and KQs relevant to current clinical practice in VA. Scope as defined by KQs is appropriate and clinically relevant. Methods are rigorous, transparent, and accomplished according to latest accepted principles of evidence based medicine.	Thank you for your confidence in our process.
2	Yes, and no comments from reviewer 2.	Thank you.
3	Yes, and no comments from reviewer 3.	Thank you.
Question 2: Is there any indication of bias in our synthesis of the evidence?		
1	No. No bias detected. Transparency of methods allows for an open assessment of bias and allows reader to assess validity and accept results as valid for use in informing clinical practice.	Thank you again for your confidence in our process.
2	No, and no comments from reviewer 2.	Thank you.
3	No. No bias detected.	Thank you.
Question 3: Are there any published or unpublished studies that we may have overlooked?		
1	No. No additional references to suggest.	Thank you.
2	No, and no comments from reviewer 2.	Thank you.
3	No – Not that I am aware of	Thank you.
Question 4: Please write additional suggestions or comments below. If applicable, please indicate the page and line numbers from the draft report.		
1	1) Could improve transparency regarding conflict of interest if: a. Drugs in this report made by manufacturers Dr Ortel has potential conflicts of interest with are identified and b. The sections Dr Ortel worked on were listed. Reader would be better able to assess bias.	We added a description of Dr. Ortel's role in the project.
1	2) Page 1 executive summary, 3rd paragraph, last sentence discussing 'Disadvantages of newer oral anticoagulants…' 'From a clinical standpoint we are most concerned with veteran safety and the lack of specific antidote is a primary concern. Would edit that sentence to place this concern first.	The recommended change has been made.
1	3) The contemporary 35-day rate of symptomatic VTE w/o prophylaxis of 4.3% (page 1); Baseline risk estimates for LMWH of 9 per 1000 symptomatic DVT, nonfatal PE 3 per 1000, mortality 3 per 1000 and major bleeding of 7 per 1000 (page 2) are extremely useful numbers for the busy clinician to know for counseling patients, comparing with treatment with NOACs (pg 4) and for making treatment decisions. Would include these numbers in the conclusions section on page 9.	We added data on the rate of VTE to the conclusion section. We did not repeat the absolute risk reductions as this information is already contained in two locations: in the bullet points and in the summary of evidence table. We will be sure that this information is contained in the VA e-brief.

52

Reviewer	Comment	Response
1	4) Page 9 Conclusion section: a). first paragraph, as noted above in #3 would put in reduced risk or increase risk numbers and b). Last paragraph… 'Based on current evidence, newer anticoagulants—particularly Xa inhibitors—are a reasonable option for thromboprophylaxis…' Agree from this evidence synthesis that Xa inhibitors are a reasonable option. Any suggested sequence of treatment? LMWH first then Xa? Or is Xa first just as reasonable as LMWH? Is there a way to assess the value of 4 per 1000 decrease in symptomatic DVT vs an increase of 2 major bleeds per 1000 treated with a Xa?	Although there are formal methods to consider multiple outcomes to develop a rank order of interventions, none of these methods are robust. The decision whether to use thromboprophylaxis, and the particular mode, is one that involves tradeoffs between potential benefits and harms. Clinicians must consider the patient's particular risks, values, and preferences when making this decision. Our data inform this decision.
1	5) 5 Page 12 3rd paragraph: 'Dabigatran etexilate is an oral reversible DTI…' Reversible seems to imply there is an antidote for reversal and there is no antidote (other than stopping the medication and letting it wear off). Recommend striking word 'reversible'.	The recommended change has been made.
1	6) Page 14 Search Strategy first paragraph: Might be more explicit as why a synthesis of high quality reviews would be more effective approach to summarizing the evidence than a perhaps a 'more standard' approach of searching the literature for RCTs and combining those in an evidence synthesis. Also, why limit the search only as far back as 1 Jan 2009. What is the rationale for the search timeframe?	We added a justification for this approach as follows: "This approach is particularly useful when different intervention options or outcomes are evaluated in multiple recent reviews and when the audience is policymakers."
1	7) Page 24 Participant Characteristics: Discussion regarding no Veterans studied in the trials and the participants were predominantly female 50-75%. Given the available evidence is there or are there any reason(s) to believe Veterans would respond differently to these treatments or wouldn't be applicable to Veterans patients? If so why? If not why not?	The applicability of the results to Veteran patients is discussion in the Applicability section of the Discussion.
1	8) Page 26 Oral Xa Inhibitors compared to LMWH: a reader might assume that all of these drugs are available in the US. While we are considering all the individual drugs, would improve transparency if drugs not available in the US were identified.	This detail has been added. Only rivaroxaban is currently available in the United States.
1	9) Page 27, paragraph 3, first sentence "In subgroup analysis, higher doses of Xa inhibitors, but not intermediate or lower doses, …" would list the doses considered high, intermediate or low in parentheses like on page 32.	The authors did not report the doses categorized as high, intermediate, or low. However, they do give the doses studied in the individual trials and we have added the dosing ranges for apixaban and rivaroxaban, drugs approved in Canada and the United States, respectively.
1	10) Page 29 Other Comparisons of Interest section, 2nd paragraph 'Low molecular weight heparin vs vitamin K antagonists, 3rd line, would put in dose regimen of enoxaparin (logiparin not available in US, so could omit dose). Same page, section immediately below 'Oral FXa inhibitors vs unfractionated heparin would list doses of fondaparinux and unfractionated heparin.	We added the dose of enoxaparin (30 mg subcutaneously every 12 hours). Fondaparinux and unfractionated heparin were evaluated in an observational study that did not report doses.

Reviewer	Comment	Response
1	11) Page 31 paragraph under 'Key Points' discussion of SRs and quality notes the industry sponsored network meta-analysis (Cohen 2012, ref 36) was rated **fair** quality. Then notes "The latter review did not provide an adequate description or quality assessment of the included trials and did not test the assumption of a constant treatment effect across different study populations--an assumption inherent to network meta-analysis." Page 32 same meta-analysis is being discussed and notes 'the composite outcomes are suspect because they combine events (composite VTE[any DVT, PE, death] and major bleeding[major, clinically relevant and minor bleeding) that have very different clinical importance'. These seem to be fatal deficiencies but the rating is **fair**. Appendix D pg 54 notes the quality rating scale and Pg 55 notes the individual trial assessments. Item 12 for the study in question (Cohen 2012, ref 36) is answered "Can't Tell" for which there is no provision in the scoring system which notes if item 12 is 'Yes' then study could be rated good or fair and if 'No' then Poor. A poor rating would have been excluded this trial from the analysis. The summary Table D-1 lists no answers for 6 of the remaining 11 items including critical items 7 and 8 which the text notes that the review is likely to have major flaws. Should the rating really be 'poor' and this analysis excluded?	We re-reviewed our quality rating for the Cohen study. We agree that it is poor quality and have excluded it from the final report.
1	12) Page 37 'Guidelines' section, First paragraph, end o paragraph notes ACCP recommends LMWH in absence of bleeding risk. Does ACCP suggest any sequence if there is an elevated bleeding risk?	We have added the ACCP recommendation for patients at increased bleeding risk: "For patients with increased bleeding risk, ACCP recommends intermittent pneumatic compression device or no prophylaxis."
1	13) Page 39 'Applicability'. End of paragraph notes private sector vs VA patients potential differences 9 (see comment #7 above). What should the reader conclude? This is a solid evidence synthesis but not applicable to VA patients? Or is applicable to VA patients?	We revised this section to state that the results likely apply to Veteran populations. We add a specific caution about higher comorbidities in Veterans, increasing the risk of bleeding.
1	14) Page 40 'Conclusion': Same comments as #4 above as this section also appears on page 9 in the Executive Summary.	As stated above, we think these data should be used to make individualized decisions with patients about the choice and mode of thromboprophylaxis.
1	15) Page 53 Appendix D, item 8, 2nd to last line '...If only qualitative analyses are completed, the study show describe...' Change 'show' to 'should'.	Thank you for noting this error. It has been corrected.
1	16) Glossary: Fantastic descriptions of confidence interval and statistical significance!	Thank you.
2	I was somewhat surprised to see the evidence that newer anticoagulants did not offer much advantage other than ease of administration and less monitoring but also troubled to see the incidence of side effects	Acknowledged

Comparative Effectiveness of New Oral Anticoagulants for Thromboprophylaxis
Evidence-based Synthesis Program

Reviewer	Comment	Response
3	Not the focus of this review, but might note that earlier this month the FDA approved rivaroxaban for treatment of deep vein thrombosis or pulmonary embolism, and to reduce the risk of recurrent DVT and PE following initial treatment. These are 2 other important clinical scenarios.	The role of newer anticoagulants for treatment of DVT and PE was reviewed in an earlier VA ESP report.
Question 5: Are there any VA clinical performance measures, programs, quality improvement measures, patient care services, or conferences that will be directly affected by this report? If so, please provide detail?		
1	There may be some inpatient performance measure for DVT prophylaxis that could be affected. Performance measure Technical Manual would need to be checked	We will ask that this report be sent to the VA clinical guideline and performance measure groups.
2	Not that I know of	Thank you.
3	No Comment???	Thank you.
Question 6: Please provide any recommendations on how this report can be revised to more directly address or assist implementation needs.		
1	See comments noted above.	Thank you.
2	N/A	Thank you.
3	It seems, at least from my perspective, that most VA providers are unaware of these reports, and fewer actually take the time to read them. However, I find that they are a valuable resource and reference tool.	Thank you.
Question 7: Please provide us with contact details of any additional individuals/stakeholders who should be made aware of this report.		
1	Lisa Longo PharmD who is PBM contact for these medications. Lisa.longo@va.gov based at VA Pittsburg	Thank you; the report has been sent to Dr. Longo, and she is one of our stakeholders in the product.
2	PBM; Chiefs of Medicine; Chief Medical Officers; Chiefs of Staff	Thank you.
3	No comments??	Thank you.

APPENDIX F. GLOSSARY

Abstract screening
The stage in a systematic review during which titles and abstracts of articles identified in the literature search are screened for inclusion or exclusion based on established criteria. Articles that pass the abstract screening stage are promoted to the full-text review stage.

Anticoagulant agents
A class of medication that prevents coagulation (blood clotting).

ClinicalTrials.gov
A registry and results database of federally and privately supported clinical trials conducted in the United States and around the world. ClinicalTrials.gov provides information about a trial's purpose, location, and participant characteristics among other details.

Cochrane Database of Systematic Reviews
A bibliographic database of peer-reviewed systematic reviews and protocols prepared by the Cochrane Review Groups in The Cochrane Collaboration.

Companion article
A publication from a trial that is not the article containing the main results of that trial. It may be a methods paper, a report of subgroup analyses, a report of combined analyses, or other auxiliary topic that adds information to the interpretation of the main publication.

Confidence interval (CI)
The range in which a particular result (such as a laboratory test) is likely to occur for everyone who has a disease. "Likely" usually means 95 percent of the time. Clinical research studies are conducted on only a certain number of people with a disease rather than all the people who have the disease. The study's results are true for the people who were in the study but not necessarily for everyone who has the disease. The CI is a statistical estimate of how much the study findings would vary if other different people participated in the study. A CI is defined by two numbers, one lower than the result found in the study and the other higher than the study's result. The size of the CI is the difference between these two numbers.

Data abstraction
The stage of a systematic review that involves a pair of trained researchers extracting reported findings specific to the research questions from the full-text articles that met the established inclusion criteria. These data form the basis of the evidence synthesis.

Deep vein thrombosis (DVT)
A blood clot that develops in the deep veins of the legs.

Direct thrombin inhibitors (DTIs)
A new class of anticoagulants that bind directly to thrombin and block its interaction with its substrates.

DistillerSR
An online application designed specifically for the screening and data extraction phases of a systematic review.

Embase
The Excerpta Medica database (EMBASE) produced by Elsevier, a major biomedical and pharmaceutical database indexing over 3500 international journals in the following fields: drug research, pharmacology, pharmaceutics, toxicology, clinical and experimental human medicine, health policy and management, public health, occupational health, environmental health, drug dependence and abuse, psychiatry, forensic medicine, and biomedical engineering or instrumentation. There is selective coverage for nursing, dentistry, veterinary medicine, psychology, and alternative medicine.

Exclusion criteria
The criteria, or standards, set out before a study or review. Exclusion criteria are used to determine whether a person should participate in a research study or whether an individual study should be excluded in a systematic review. Exclusion criteria may include age, previous treatments, and other medical conditions.

Factor Xa (FXa) inhibitor
A new class of anticoagulants that bind directly to factor Xa and block its interaction with other substrates.

Full-text review
The stage of a systematic review in which a pair of trained researches evaluates the full-text of study articles for potential inclusion in the review.

GRADE
Grading of Recommendations Assessment, Development, and Evaluation (GRADE), a system of assessing the quality of medical evidence and evaluating the strength of recommendations based on the evidence.

Inclusion criteria
The criteria, or standards, set out before the systematic review. Inclusion criteria are used to determine whether an individual study can be included in a systematic review. Inclusion criteria may include population, study design, sex, age, type of disease being treated, previous treatments, and other medical conditions.

Low molecular weight heparin
A class of medication used to treat thrombosis or for prophylaxis in situations that lead to a high risk of thrombosis. These medications have a more predictable anticoagulant response than naturally occurring unfractionated heparin.

Optimal information size
The number of patients that need to be included in a pooled analysis (meta-analysis) to provide sufficient power to detect the smallest clinically important difference in treatment effect.

PRISMA
Preferred Reporting Items for Systematic Reviews and Meta-Analyses, an evidence-based minimum set of items for reporting in systematic reviews and meta-analyses.

Publication bias
The tendency of researchers to publish experimental findings that have a positive result, while not publishing the findings when the results are negative or inconclusive. The effect of publication bias is that published studies may be misleading. When information that differs from that of the published study is not known, people are able to draw conclusions using only information from the published studies.

PubMed®
A database of citations for biomedical literature from MEDLINE®, life science journals, and online books in the fields of medicine, nursing, dentistry, veterinary medicine, the health care system, and preclinical sciences.

Pulmonary embolism (PE)
Blocking of the pulmonary artery (lungs) or one of its branches by a clot.

Randomized controlled trial
A prospective, analytical, experimental study using primary data generated in the clinical environment. Individuals similar at the beginning of the trial are randomly allocated to two or more treatment groups and the outcomes the groups are compared after sufficient followup time. Properly executed, the RCT is the strongest evidence of the clinical efficacy of preventive and therapeutic procedures in the clinical setting.

Risk
A way of expressing the chance that something will happen. It is a measure of the association between exposure to something and what happens (the outcome). Risk is the same as probability, but it usually is used to describe the probability of an adverse event. It is the rate of events (such as breast cancer) in the total population of people who could have the event (such as women of a certain age).

Statistical significance
A mathematical technique to measure whether the results of a study are likely to be true. Statistical significance is calculated as the probability that an effect observed in a research study is occurring because of chance. Statistical significance is usually expressed as a P-value. The smaller the P-value, the less likely it is that the results are due to chance (and more likely that the results are true). Researchers generally believe the results are probably true if the statistical significance is a P-value less than 0.05 ($p<.05$).

Strength of evidence (SOE)
A measure of how confident reviewers are about decisions that may be made based on a body of evidence. SOE is evaluated using one of four grades: (1) *High* confidence that the evidence reflects the true effect; further research is very unlikely to change reviewer confidence in the estimate of effect; (2) *moderate* confidence that the evidence reflects the true effect; further research may change the confidence in the estimate of effect and may change the estimate; (3) *low* confidence that the evidence reflects the true effect; further research is likely to change the confidence in the estimate of effect and is likely to change the estimate; and (4) *insufficient*; the evidence either is unavailable or does not permit a conclusion.

Systematic review
A summary of the clinical literature. A systematic review is a critical assessment and evaluation of all research studies that address a particular clinical issue. The researchers use an organized method of locating, assembling, and evaluating a body of literature on a particular topic using a set of specific criteria. A systematic review typically includes a description of the findings of the collection of research studies. The systematic review may also include a quantitative pooling of data, called a meta-analysis.

Venous thromboembolism (VTE)
Obstruction of a vein or veins (embolism) by a blood clot (thrombus) in the blood stream; includes deep vein thrombosis (DVT) and pulmonary embolism (PE).

Vitamin K antagonist (warfarin)
An anticoagulant that acts by inhibiting the synthesis of vitamin K-dependent coagulation factors; i.e., I, VII, IX and X.